great international diabetic desserts

Karin Cadwell, Ph.D., R.N.

Foreword by Bruce Mirvis, M.D., F.A.A.P.

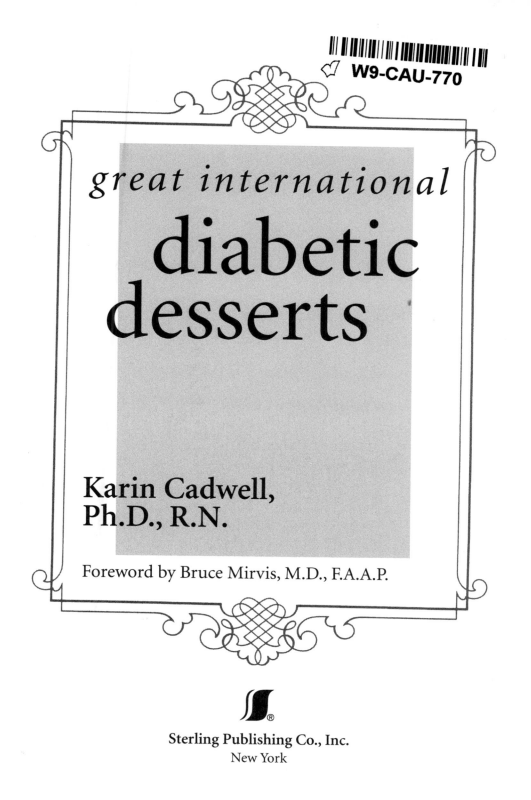

Sterling Publishing Co., Inc.
New York

Library of Congress Cataloging-in-Publication Data

Cadwell, Karin.
    Great international diabetic desserts / Karin Cadwell ; foreword by Bruce Mirvis.
        p. cm.
    Includes index.
    ISBN 0-8069-1889-6
    1. Diabetes—Diet therapy recipes. 2. Desserts. I. Title.
    RC662.C3163   1999
    641.5'6413—dc21   99-20752
                                                       CIP

10 9 8 7 6 5 4 3 2 1

Published by Sterling Publishing Company, Inc.
387 Park Avenue South, New York, N.Y. 10016
© 1999 by Karin Cadwell
Distributed in Canada by Sterling Publishing
C/o Canadian Manda Group, One Atlantic Avenue, Suite 105
Toronto, Ontario, Canada M6K 3E7
Distributed in Great Britain and Europe by Cassell PLC
Wellington House, 125 Strand, London WC2R 0BB, England
Distributed in Australia by Capricorn Link (Australia) Pty Ltd.
P.O. Box 6651, Baulkham Hills, Business Centre, NSW 2153, Australia
Manufactured in the United States
All rights reserved

Sterling ISBN 0-8069-1889-6

Contents

Foreword

Juvenile diabetes has a tremendous impact on the lives of individuals who are affected, as well as on their families. It has certainly impacted our family; we have two children who have juvenile onset diabetes.

I vividly remember the day when our child's physician told us that our three-year-old son had diabetes. I am a pediatrician and my wife is a nurse, so we should have been prepared for this information. However, we definitely were not. We understood the pathophysiology of juvenile onset diabetes mellitus; what we did not know and were not prepared to deal with was what having a child with diabetes would mean to him and our family. Four years later our nine-year-old daughter was diagnosed with diabetes also. We were no more prepared for this news, but we were better educated about the nuances of living with children who have special needs. As they have grown and matured, our son, now 22, and daughter, now 24, have remained very close. They are involved in teaching their peers with and without diabetes about how to eat a healthy diet and live with diabetes. Our son is a fireman and medic; our daughter, who is happily married, is a pre-school teacher.

Our initial thoughts of what we could feed our sickly 3-year-old were indeed overwhelming. How do you tell a child he can never have a birthday cake or ice cream or eat like everybody else while on vacation? We looked to our community for help and found little support or guidance. So we went to work and helped organize a diabetes support group to help educate not only ourselves, but also other families that had children with diabetes.

I often refer to diabetes as a "hidden disease," because it doesn't have the physical stigma of cerebral palsy, the horror of leukemia, or the emaciation of cystic fibrosis. I once informed a family that their child had both diabetes and leukemia. His parents and extended family could focus only on the diagnosis of leukemia. I explained that in three years, when the leukemia was cured, he would still have diabetes, a lifelong disease. When I last heard from him, he had graduated from college and had a family of his own. His leukemia was completely cured. He continues, however, to cope with keeping his diabetes under good control.

Educating our family, friends, schools, and places of employment about juvenile onset diabetes remains a never-ending challenge. Our son was the only person in his school with diabetes. Once he had the school bus driver stop the bus, because our son said his blood sugar was low and he needed gum to raise his blood sugar. The driver was so nervous about having a diabetic child on the bus, he would have done anything our son asked him to do. The driver stopped and bought him sugarless gum. We didn't know whether to be angry at our son for manipulating the system or pleased at his ingenuity; we didn't know whether to praise the bus driver for being so responsive or challenge him for being so gullible. We had no idea how to explain to our friends that this sort of behavior was not funny. Few people understand the seriousness of low blood sugar; even fewer are aware that children with chronic illnesses can be inappropriately manipulative of the people around them.

Several things have emerged from living with diabetes for 19 years. Foremost among them, children are children first, no matter what their diagnosis or medical limitations. Our daughter made this point very clear to us. She emphasized that rewards came in many forms besides candy. While experiencing new situations, children need affection, cuddling, and help much more than they do the immediate gratification of a piece of candy.

Finding the ultimate cure for juvenile diabetes is an important goal. Members of our family have dedicated the past 19 years to finding a cure for diabetes, and our zeal is unrelenting in seeking ways to educate children with diabetes, as well as their parents and the public. Because of the efforts of my family and so many others the prospect of a cure for juvenile diabetes in the near future is a real possibility.

Being a child with diabetes is more difficult than having children with diabetes. We always allowed our children to live lives as normal as possible. Doing so required a good deal of planning and education. We adjusted their insulin, not what they were excluded from eating, when they went to parties. For school parties, we brought cupcakes, half of them without icing; and diet soda was always available. Yes, there was some cheating; those ever-present candy wrappers in the bed. Over time our children learned to control their cravings and with maturity learned to eat nutritious foods and limit free sugars and fats. Occasional straying from a rigidly controlled diet is inevitable, but with support and patience these occurrences can be minimized. We have continued to be advocates, to remind parents to give their children a healthy, balanced diet. Cookbooks with such great recipes and suggestions as Karin Cadwell's makes the task of preparing nutritious desserts much easier.

—*Bruce Mirvis, M.D., F.A.A.P.*

Introduction

Those of you who have read the introductions to my previous diabetic dessert cookbooks, *Great Diabetic Desserts & Sweets* and *Diabetic Sweet Treats*, know that my underlying philosophy is that desserts for people on diabetic diets should be so delicious and beautiful that they can be served to everyone! Diabetic desserts are, after all, lower in fat, sugar, and cholesterol than comparable treats and are not any less tasty.

My strong feelings about not having lesser choices for people on diabetic diets began when I was a teenager and noticed that dessert for my newly diagnosed diabetic uncle Tom was often an afterthought. I remember my mother and her friends priding themselves on their fancy dessert recipes for dinner parties, but dessert for Uncle Tom was often a last-minute scramble.

Then my grandfather was also diagnosed with diabetes, and my grandmother took his diet very seriously, making special desserts for him and bringing them along wrapped in waxed paper when they went out.

Things have changed in the past few years. On the one hand, diabetic diets have become less complicated and less restricted. On the other hand, people without a need to adhere to a diet because of a diagnosed medical problem are choosing to eat healthier foods and follow diets that have less sugar. The desserts in this book are nutritious and delicious for your whole family and all your guests.

One thing you'll notice right away is that I use sugar as a sweetener rather than relying on substitutes. That's possible because I've chosen "Old World" recipes that don't rely on sugar for taste. It's possible to replace the eggs with egg substitute in many of these recipes; I've indicated it in the recipe wherever it's appropriate, but the cholesterol per serving is based on the use of eggs. Butter, margarine, and the new fat-free butter and oil replacement can be used interchangeably in almost every recipe, but again, the calorie, fat, and cholesterol analyses have been calculated based on the use of butter. If you do use margarine, be sure to use the stick type. Tub margarine, especially "light" margarine, won't work in most recipes.

The theme of this book is traditional desserts from various cultures. In my research one thing I noticed was how many cultures prized the same ingredients—apples, raisins, milk, eggs, and flour! The variations are endless and charming.

I developed recipes that are fairly easy to make and that require no special skills or fancy equipment. While a food processor or blender may be called for in a recipe, it is possible to achieve similar results with a little extra time and effort, by cutting finely with a knife. The recipes don't call for hard-to-find ingredients, either. A few recipes *are* time-consuming, involving soaking dough overnight or letting it rise overnight, but they're well worth the time and effort. The directions let you know how long a recipe will take and if there's a time-consuming step or two.

Working on the recipes for this book was a heartwarming experience for me. I felt a special connection to women in kitchens around the world, taking ordinary ingredients to make special desserts for their families and guests. It's my hope that as you prepare them you'll feel that same appreciation for their skill and ingenuity. Happy cooking. Eat in good health.

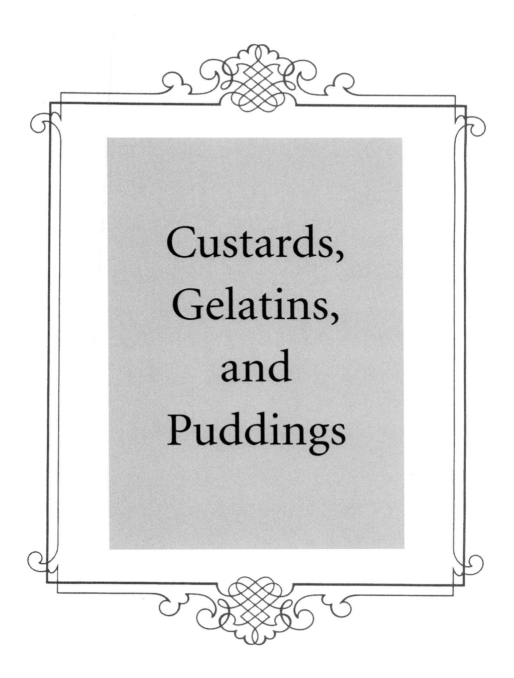

Custards, Gelatins, and Puddings

Middle Eastern Ashoura Dessert

My daughter Kajsa and granddaughter Emma love this simple Middle Eastern traditional dessert.

½ C or 1 lb.	barley	125 mL
	water	
½ C	lowfat 1% milk	125 mL
1 pinch	cinnamon, or other flavoring	1 pinch

Wash and rinse the barley and soak it in plenty of water for about 10 minutes. Drain, rinse again, and place in a saucepan. Add enough water to cover with an extra inch (3 cm). Cook for at least two hours. The grains will swell and burst. Transfer them to a bowl. Cool completely. Cover the bowl tightly with aluminum foil or plastic wrap. Refrigerate until ready to serve. This can be enjoyed at any temperature.

Fill a bowl with *ashoura* and hot or cold milk, according to taste. Sprinkle with ground cinnamon or other flavoring.

Yield: 16 servings.
Each serving contains:

Calories (Kcal): 105
Carbohydrates (g): 22
Sodium (mg): 7
Diabetic exchange: 1 starch

Total fat (g): 1
Protein (g): 4
Cholesterol (mg): 0

Indian Semolina Halva

You can buy semolina at a health food store or specialty food store. You are looking for the grain, not semolina flour.

5 T	vegetable oil or clarified butter	75 mL
3 T	slivered almonds	45 mL
2 C	semolina, uncooked	500 mL
½ C	sugar	125 mL
1¼ C	water, boiling	310 mL
3 T	golden raisins	45 mL
¼ t	cardamom seeds, finely crushed	2 mL

Heat the vegetable oil over medium heat in a large, heavy-bottomed frying pan. Add the almonds. Stir and remove when golden. Drain on paper towels. Put the semolina into the oil and sauté over low heat, stirring until the semolina turns golden brown. Stir in the sugar. Slowly add the boiling water while stirring. Cook over low heat for 5–7 minutes. Stir in the raisins and cardamom. Stir and cook for another 5 minutes. Serve hot or warm.

Yield: 12 servings.
Each serving contains:
Calories (Kcal): 210.9   Total fat (g): 7.0
Carbohydrates (g): 33.5   Protein (g): 3.7
Sodium (mg): 2   Cholesterol (mg): 0
Diabetic exchange: 1 starch; ½ fat

Mexican Bread Pudding

This bread pudding is a traditional dessert of the Mexican Lenten season.

4 slices	white bread, toasted and cubed	4 slices
3 C	lowfat 1% milk, scalded	750 mL
½ C	brown sugar	125 mL
1 t	nutmeg	5 mL
1½ t	cinnamon	8 mL
1 pinch	salt	1 pinch
3 whole	eggs, well beaten	3 whole
¼ C	butter, margarine, or fat-free replacement, melted	60 mL
1 t	vanilla extract	5 mL
¼ C	seedless raisins	60 mL
3 oz.	fat-free cream cheese, cubed	85 g

Combine bread cubes and scalded milk in a greased two-quart (2 L) baking dish; let stand for 10 minutes. In a mixing bowl, combine the sugar, spices, and salt. Add the eggs and melted butter, and mix in the rest of the ingredients. Pour over the bread cubes. Stir lightly to blend. Bake for 30 minutes in a preheated 350° F (180° C) oven.

Yield: 8 servings.
Each serving contains:
Calories (Kcal): 210   Total fat (g): 9
Carbohydrates (g): 25   Protein (g): 7
Sodium (mg): 264   Cholesterol (mg): 101
Diabetic exchange: 1 whole milk; 1 fruit

Polish Black Bread Pudding

Use your blender to make bread crumbs from pumpernickel for this recipe. The more flavorful the bread, the better the pudding.

6 whole	eggs, separated	6 whole
6 T	sugar	90 mL
1 C	pumpernickel bread crumbs	250 mL
	cinnamon, to taste	
¼ t	ground cloves	2 mL
1 T	butter, margarine, or fat-free replacement, melted	15 mL
1 t	bread crumbs	5 mL

Beat the egg whites until stiff. In another bowl, gently blend the egg yolks and sugar. Add bread crumbs, cinnamon, cloves, and the melted butter. Mix thoroughly and fold in the stiffly beaten egg whites. Line buttered pan with bread crumbs and pour in the mixture. Bake in 350° F (180° C) oven for 25 to 30 minutes.

Yield: 8 servings.
Each serving contains:
Calories (Kcal): 160
Carbohydrates (g): 20
Sodium (mg): 158
Total fat (g): 6
Protein (g): 6
Cholesterol (mg): 163
Diabetic exchange: ½ starch; ½ fat

German Rye Bread and Apple Pudding

I made this using dark rye bread. Whitney Mirvis was visiting the first time I made this, and she and I couldn't believe how fabulous it tasted. These simple ingredients add up to a really great pudding.

11 slices	pumpernickel bread, cubed	11 slices
1 C	unsweetened apple juice	250 mL
1½ C	dry white wine	375 mL
1½ lbs.	green apples, peeled, cored, and thickly sliced	680 g
5 T	sugar	75 mL
½ t	cinnamon	3 mL
½ C	raisins	125 mL
4 T	butter, margarine, or fat-free replacement	60 mL

Put two-thirds of the bread cubes into a bowl and pour the apple juice and wine over them. Stir. Place a thick layer of the bread cubes on the bottom of a well-greased casserole. Add a layer of apples. Sprinkle with sugar and cinnamon. Continue layering until the apples are used up. Sprinkle the raisins on top of the apples and top with the remaining bread. Dot with the butter. Bake in a 400° F (200° C) oven for 45 minutes. Serve warm.

Yield: 10 servings.
Each serving contains:

Calories (Kcal): 215	Total fat (g): 65
Carbohydrates (g): 35	Protein (g): 3
Sodium (mg): 223	Cholesterol (mg): 15

Diabetic exchange: 1 starch; 1 fruit; 1 fat

Finnish Whipped Berry Pudding

You can't imagine the color, volume, and taste when this whips up.

3 C	cranberry juice, low-calorie	750 mL
2 T	sugar	30 mL
½ C	Cream of Wheat, uncooked	125 mL
1 t	raspberry extract	5 mL

In a 1½- to 2-quart (1½ to 2 L) saucepan, bring the cranberry juice to a boil over moderate heat. Add the sugar, a little at a time, to the boiling juice, then slowly add the Cream of Wheat, stirring briskly with a wooden spoon. Reduce the heat and simmer for 6 to 8 minutes, stirring occasionally, until the mixture becomes a thick purée.

Using a rubber spatula, transfer the purée to a large mixing bowl. Beat at the highest speed of an electric mixer for 10 to 15 minutes, or until the pudding has doubled in volume, turned a delicate pink, and is light and fluffy. Beat in the raspberry extract. Pour into individual dessert bowls. Serve immediately.

Yield: 12 servings.
Each serving contains:

Calories (Kcal): 46	Total fat (g): 0
Carbohydrates (g): 10	Protein (g): 1
Sodium (mg): 2	Cholesterol (mg): 0
Diabetic exchange: 1 fruit	

English Fresh Strawberry Pudding

Early English settlers found the strawberries in Virginia four times bigger than the ones they remembered from their homes in England.

2 C	fresh strawberries, washed and hulled	500 mL
2 T	sugar	30 mL
	water	
2 pkgs. (3 oz. each)	sugar-free strawberry flavored gelatin	170 g
4 C	low-fat frozen non-dairy whipped topping	1 L

In a small bowl, crush the strawberries with a fork. Sprinkle with the sugar. Mix, cover, and let stand for an hour. Drain the juice, reserving it in a measuring cup. Add enough water to make 1½ cups (375 mL) of liquid. In a small saucepan, bring the liquid to a boil. Stir in the gelatin. Remove from heat. Stir until the gelatin dissolves. Let cool, then pour the gelatin over the strawberries. Stir. Fold the whipped topping into the strawberry mixture. Transfer to a soufflé dish or other serving dish. Refrigerate for several hours before serving.

Yield: 10 servings.
Each serving contains:
Calories (Kcal): 71.8
Carbohydrates (g): 11
Sodium (mg): 76
Diabetic exchange: 1 fruit

Total fat (g): 0.1
Protein (g): 0.4
Cholesterol (mg): 0

German Black Forest Cherry Pudding

You can replace the Kirschwasser with water and cherry extract. The flavor won't be as authentic, but it's still very good.

½ lb.	small, sweet cherries, stemmed and pitted	225 g
⅓ C	sugar	90 mL
2 T	Kirschwasser liqueur	30 mL
4 T	unsalted butter, margarine, or fat-free replacement	60 mL
6 T	all-purpose flour	90 mL
1¼ C	lowfat 1% milk	310 mL
3	eggs, separated, extra large	3
⅛ t	salt	1 mL

Put the cherries in a bowl with 1 T (15 mL) sugar and the Kirschwasser. With the back of a spoon, crush the cherries against the side of the bowl, macerating them and mixing them with the sugar and Kirschwasser. Melt the butter in a heavy saucepan over moderate heat. Using a whisk, blend in the flour. Add the milk and remaining sugar and cook for 3 to 5 minutes, stirring constantly, until thickened and smooth. Put the egg yolks in a small bowl and mix well. While stirring, gradually add a cup of the hot milk mixture to the egg yolks. Blend this mixture back into the saucepan and mix well. Add the cherries and the liquid in the bowl to the milk mixture. Mix well. Beat the egg whites until they are stiff. Stir about one-quarter of the beaten whites into the cherry mixture to lighten it, then gently but thoroughly fold in the balance. Pour into a 2½- to 3-quart (2½ to 3 liter) well-greased soufflé dish and bake immediately in a 350° F (180° C) preheated oven for 40 to 45 minutes, until puffed and browned and until the mixture quivers when you nudge the dish. Serve immediately.

Yield: 6 servings.
Each serving contains:
Calories (Kcal): 230
Carbohydrates (g): 24
Sodium (mg): 103
Total fat (g): 11
Protein (g): 6
Cholesterol (mg): 130
Diabetic exchange: 1 starch; 1 fruit; 2 fats

British Queen of Puddings

This baked pudding has a meringue "crown"—that's why it's the queen!

1 whole	lemon peel	1 whole
2 C	lowfat 1% milk	500 mL
2 T	butter	30 mL
¼ C	sugar	60 mL
1 C	fresh white-bread crumbs (remove crust, pulverize in a blender or processor, or fork-shred)	250 mL
3 large	egg yolks	3 large
3 large	egg whites	3 large
2 T	sugar	30 mL
¼ C	all-fruit raspberry jam	60 mL

Put the lemon peel and milk in a heavy saucepan over a low heat and simmer for 4 or 5 minutes. Discard the peel. Add the butter and sugar, increase the heat, and cook, stirring constantly, until the sugar dissolves. Remove from heat. Stir in the bread crumbs and set aside to cool. Preheat the oven to 350° F (180° C). Beat in the egg yolks. Pour the mixture into a well-greased pie pan. Smooth the top. Bake for 20 minutes. The pudding will be firm. Set aside to cool. Beat the egg whites until they foam. Add the remaining sugar and beat until the egg whites form stiff peaks. Melt the jam over low heat in a small saucepan. Pour the jam over the top of the cool pudding. Spread the egg whites over the jam. Return to the oven and bake for 10 to 12 minutes. The top will be golden brown.

Yield: 8 servings.
Each serving contains:

Calories (Kcal): 199	Total fat (g): 8
Carbohydrates (g): 26	Protein (g): 5
Sodium (mg): 115	Cholesterol (mg): 90

Diabetic exchange: 1 starch; 1 fruit; 1 fat

Polish Kutia Pudding

This is a traditional Christmas pudding.

3 C	water	750 mL
⅔ C	wheat cereal, such as farina or Cream of Wheat	175 mL
1 C	water	250 mL
2 T	poppy seeds	30 mL
⅔ C	raisins	30 mL
½ C	walnuts, chopped	125 mL
½ C	honey	125 mL
¼ C	slivered almonds	60 mL
1 t	vanilla	5 mL
½ C	low-fat frozen non-dairy whipped topping	125 mL

Put the water into a saucepan and bring to a boil. Slowly stir in the cereal and mix so there are no lumps. Cook, covered, in an oven under low heat for one hour, stirring occasionally. Remove from heat. The water should be absorbed. Meanwhile heat the one cup (250 mL) of water and the poppy seeds in a small saucepan until the poppy seeds are soft, about 10 minutes. Drain. In a serving bowl combine the cooked cereal, drained poppy seeds, raisins, walnuts, honey, almonds, and vanilla. Chill. Serve topped with a dollop of whipped topping.

Yield: 12 servings
Each serving contains:
Calories (Kcal): 165   Total fat (g): 5.3
Carbohydrates (g): 27.9   Protein (g): 3.5
Sodium (mg): 6   Cholesterol (mg): 0
Diabetic exchange: 2 starch

Swedish Rum Pudding

If you'd rather not use rum, substitute half a cup of milk and a teaspoon of rum extract.

1 env.	gelatin	1 env.
¼ C	cold water	60 mL
5 large	egg yolks, beaten	5 large
½ C	sugar	125 mL
2 C	hot lowfat 1% milk	500 mL
½ C	rum	125 mL
1 C	low-fat frozen non-dairy whipped topping	250 mL

Soak the gelatin in the cold water until soft. Beat the egg yolks with the sugar until frothy and lemon-colored, then slowly add the hot milk, stirring constantly. Pour the mixture into the top of a double boiler, over boiling water, and cook for a few minutes until smooth and creamy. Add the gelatin mixture to this; blend well and cool.

When the cream is cool, add the rum and the whipped topping. Serve in six dessert dishes.

Yield: 6 servings.
Each serving contains:

Calories (Kcal): 219	Total fat (g): 5
Carbohydrates (g): 25	Protein (g): 5
Sodium (mg): 64	Cholesterol (mg): 180

Diabetic exchange: 1 lowfat milk; 1 fruit

Irish Tipsy Parson

The name says it all! Make this in the morning for an impressive dessert after dinner.

1 C	strawberries, whole (thaw if frozen)	250 mL
1 T	sugar	15 mL
½ cake	angel food cake, cubed	½ cake
3 T	sweet Sherry	45 mL
1 pkg.	sugar-free vanilla pudding mix (prepared for 4 servings)	1 pkg.
1 tsp	vanilla	5 mL
2 C	lowfat 1% milk	500 mL
1 C	low-fat frozen non-dairy whipped topping	250 mL
	additional whipped topping as garnish (optional)	
¼ C	toasted almonds (optional)	60 mL

Combine fruit and sugar in a bowl and set aside. Toss the cake cubes and Sherry in a separate bowl and set aside. Make the vanilla pudding according to package directions using the two cups of lowfat milk. Stir in the vanilla. Let the cooked pudding cool for 15 minutes. Stir in the cup of whipped topping. Layer the cake cubes, fruit, and pudding in a serving bowl or individual dishes. Refrigerate for at least four hours before serving. Decorate with whipped topping and toasted almonds, if desired.

Yield: 10 servings.
Each serving contains:
Calories (Kcal): 128   Total fat (g): 1
Carbohydrates (g): 25   Protein (g): 4
Sodium (mg): 218   Cholesterol (mg): 3
Diabetic exchange: ½ meat; 2 fruit

Irish Coffee Mold

Use a fancy gelatin mold and unmold before serving. If you use a ring mold, pile the frozen non-dairy whipped topping in the center space.

1¼ C	strong coffee	310 mL
2 T	sugar	30 mL
2 whole	cloves	2 whole
1 strip	lemon peel	1 strip
1 strip	orange peel	1 strip
1 small	cinnamon stick	1 small
1 env.	gelatin powder, unsweetened	1 env.
¼ C	Irish Mist	60 mL
1 C	low-fat frozen non-dairy whipped topping	250 mL

Combine coffee, sugar, cloves, lemon peel, orange peel, and cinnamon in a small saucepan. Bring to a boil, and boil for two minutes. Strain the mixture to remove the pieces of peel and the spices. Put the Irish Mist in a small bowl and sprinkle it with the gelatin. Stir. Add the hot-coffee mixture and stir until the gelatin is dissolved. Rinse a two-cup (500 mL) mold with cold water. Pour the gelatin mixture into the mold. Refrigerate overnight. Unmold at serving time by dipping the mold briefly into a pan of hot water. Hold a serving plate over the gelatin side of the mold tightly while inverting. Top with whipped topping.

Yield: 4 servings.
Each serving contains:
Calories (Kcal): 183   Total fat (g): 1
Carbohydrates (g): 16   Protein (g): 19
Sodium (mg): 72   Cholesterol (mg): 0
Diabetic exchange: 1½ skim milk; 1 lean meat

Madigan's Velvet Trousers

An Irish gelatin dessert. Light and lovely. I have trouble getting this to the table. The spoon marks in the surface start appearing the minute the dessert is in the refrigerator.

1 pkg.	unflavored gelatin	1 pkg.
¼ C	cold water	60 mL
2 C	low-fat frozen non-dairy whipped topping (8 oz. container)	500 mL
1½ T	clear honey	23 mL
2 T	Irish Mist	30 mL

Pour the gelatin into the top of a double boiler. Add the water and stir. Set over the bottom of a double boiler filled with gently boiling water. Stir until the gelatin dissolves. Remove the top pan from the double boiler. Slowly mix in the honey and whiskey. Mix well. Fold in the dissolved gelatin using a spatula. Spoon into four small glass serving dishes. Tightly cover the serving dishes with aluminum foil or plastic wrap. Refrigerate for several hours before serving.

Yield: 4 servings.
Each serving contains:

Calories (Kcal): 116

Carbohydrates (g): 16

Sodium (mg): 46

Diabetic exchange: 1 fruit

Total fat (g): 0

Protein (g): 1

Cholesterol (mg): 0

Italian Wine Gelatin with Fresh Fruit

Using wine in the gelatin makes for a very sophisticated flavor, but you may use non-alcoholic wine if you prefer.

2 envs.	unflavored gelatin	2 envs.
1½ C	cold water	375 mL
1½ C	dry white wine	375 mL
2 T	sugar	30 mL
¼ C	dry red wine	60 mL
1 C	blueberries	250 mL
1 C	raspberries	250 mL

Stir the gelatin and cold water together in a small saucepan. Add the white wine and the sugar. Cook over a low heat, stirring constantly, until the gelatin is dissolved. Add the red wine. Cool to room temperature. Arrange the berries in a gelatin mold or serving bowls. Add the cooled gelatin. Chill overnight.

Yield: 8 servings.
Each serving contains:

Calories (Kcal): 76

Total fat (g): 0

Carbohydrates (g): 10

Protein (g): 1

Sodium (mg): 10

Cholesterol (mg): 0

Diabetic exchange: 1 fruit

Russian Apple Kisel

This is a nice and cool warm-weather dessert. In cooler weather I serve it warm.

4 C	green apples—peeled, cored, and quartered	1 L
3 C	cold water	750 mL
⅓ C	sugar	90 mL
1 T	cornstarch	15 mL
1 T	cold water	15 mL

Place the prepared cooking apples in a pot with the 3 cups (750 mL) of cold water. Bring the water to a boil, reduce the heat, and simmer uncovered for about 10 minutes, or until the apples are tender. Drain the apples and mash them. Add the sugar and stir. Return to the cooking pot and bring to a boil.

In a teacup, dissolve the cornstarch in the tablespoon of cold water. Pour the cornstarch mixture into the fruit. Cook another 2–3 minutes, until the mixture thickens. Refrigerate before serving in individual serving dishes.

Yield: 4 servings.
Each serving contains:

Calories (Kcal): 122
Carbohydrates (g): 31
Sodium (mg): 8
Diabetic exchange: 2 fruit

Total fat (g): 0
Protein (g): 0
Cholesterol (mg): 0

Russian Apricot Kisel

Anyone who likes apricots will love this kisel. Serve it cold in warm weather or warm in cold weather. Similar to the previous recipe, yet altogether different!

1½ C	dried apricots	375 mL
3 C	water	750 mL
2 T	sugar	30 mL
1 T	cornstarch	15 mL
1 T	water	15 mL

Place the dried apricots in a pot with the 3 cups (750 mL) of cold water. Bring the water to a boil, reduce the heat, and simmer uncovered for 10 minutes or so, until the apples are tender. Drain the apricots and dice into small cubes. Add the sugar and stir. Return to the cooking pot and bring to a boil.

In a teacup, dissolve the cornstarch in the tablespoon of cold water. Pour the cornstarch mixture into the fruit. Cook another 2–3 minutes until the mixture thickens. Refrigerate before serving in individual serving dishes.

Yield: 4 servings.
Each serving contains:

Calories (Kcal): 175
Carbohydrates (g): 45
Sodium (mg): 14
Diabetic exchange: 3 fruit

Total fat (g): 0
Protein (g): 2
Cholesterol (mg): 0

Austrian Salzburg Soufflé

A classic soufflé with a fresh lemon tang.

3 large	egg yolks	3 large
1 t	vanilla extract	5 mL
½ whole	rind of lemon	½ whole
2 T	flour	30 mL
5 large	egg whites	5 large
1 pinch	salt	1 pinch
2 T	confectioner's sugar	30 mL

Beat the egg yolks with the vanilla extract, lemon peel, and flour. In a mixing bowl, combine the egg whites and salt and whip until stiff peaks begin to form. Gradually add the sugar. Beat until stiff. Gently fold the egg whites into the yolk and flour mixture. Place in a well-greased 8½-inch (21 cm) soufflé dish. With a spatula make three or four separate mounds. Bake in a preheated 350° F (180° C) oven for 15–20 minutes or until light brown on top. As with all soufflés, serve immediately.

Yield: 6 servings.
Each serving contains:

Calories (Kcal): 64	Total fat (g): 3
Carbohydrates (g): 5	Protein (g): 5
Sodium (mg): 72	Cholesterol (mg): 106

Diabetic exchange: 1 medium-fat meat

French Strawberry and Peach Soufflé

This is a foolproof soufflé, but only if you serve it right away.

2 large	peaches, ripe or canned, diced	2 large
13 oz.	small frozen strawberries, diced	370 g
⅓ C	Grand Marnier liqueur	80 g
4 large	egg yolks	4 large
2 T	confectioner's sugar	40 g
4 large	egg whites	4 large
1 pinch	salt	1 pinch

Combine the diced peaches, strawberries, and Grand Marnier and marinate for two to three hours. In a mixing bowl, cream the egg yolks and sugar until pale and creamy. Spoon the fruit and liquid into the yolk mixture. In another bowl, beat the egg whites with a pinch of salt until they are stiff. Gently fold the egg whites into the yolk mixture. Turn into four well-greased soufflé dishes. Bake in a preheated 400° F (200° C) oven approximately 15 minutes, or until they have risen and are golden brown on top. Serve immediately.

Yield: 4 servings.
Each serving contains:

Calories (Kcal): 210	Total fat (g): 6
Carbohydrates (g): 23	Protein (g): 213
Sodium (mg): 96	Cholesterol (mg): 213

Diabetic exchange: 1 medium-fat meat; 2 fruit

Greek Whole Wheat Porridge

Even people who think they don't like whole wheat might like to try this. It's very high in B vitamins and fiber.

5 C	whole wheat bulgur	1250 mL
	water	
1 pinch	cinnamon	1 pinch
1 C	almonds, coarsely ground (optional)	250 mL
½ C	dried currants (optional)	125 mL

Place the bulgur in a large saucepan. Cover with cold water and let stand overnight. Drain, then cover with fresh cold water. Simmer about four hours, or until tender, stirring frequently. Add water as needed. The stock will become very thick. Add cinnamon to taste. Stir in the almonds and/or currants, if desired. Serve hot.

Yield: 20 servings.
Each serving contains:

Calories (Kcal): 119
Carbohydrates (g): 27
Sodium (mg): 6
Diabetic exchange: 2 starch

Total fat (g): 0
Protein (g): 4
Cholesterol (mg): 0

Swedish Rice Porridge

My grandmother's rice porridge recipe! If you don't like raisins, leave them out—it's still good. The person who gets the hidden almond is the lucky one.

3 C	lowfat 1% milk	750 mL
½ C	long-grain rice	125 mL
⅓ C	raisins	80 mL
¼ t	salt	2 mL
⅓ C	sugar	80 mL
1 whole	almond, blanched	1 whole
¼ t	ground cinnamon	2 mL

In a heavy saucepan bring the milk to a boil. Stir in the rice, raisins, salt, and sugar. Cover and cook over low heat, stirring occasionally, until most of the milk is absorbed, about 30 to 45 minutes. Stir in the almond and cinnamon. Spoon into a serving dish. Serve warm.

Yield: 8 servings.
Each serving contains:

Calories (Kcal): 89	Total fat (g): 1
Carbohydrates (g): 17	Protein (g): 3
Sodium (mg): 114	Cholesterol (mg): 4
Diabetic exchange: 1 starch	

Egyptian Sutlach

A traditional pudding with a rice base and caramel glaze. It's nice to make when you're home all day.

Pudding

5 T	uncooked ground rice (grind in a blender)	75 mL
2 quarts	lowfat 1% milk	2 L
1 T	sugar	15 mL

Caramel

½ C	sugar	125 mL
¾ C	water	185 mL
1 squeeze	lemon juice	1 squeeze
½ C	water	125 mL

In a large, heavy-bottomed pan, combine the rice and just enough milk to make a smooth, thin paste. Set the pan over very low heat and stir continuously, gradually adding the additional milk and the sugar. When all the milk has been added, bring to a boil, stirring often to avoid burning the bottom, and cook until the mixture is thick and creamy. This takes an hour or more. Pour the pudding into a glass ovenproof baking dish to a depth of only between one and two inches (3–5 cm). If necessary, use two shallow pans. Preheat the oven to 300° F (150° C) while you make the caramel.

Put the sugar and ¾ cup (185 mL) water in a small saucepan. Cook over low heat, stirring, until the mixture becomes transparent. Add the squeeze of lemon juice. Turn up the heat and cook until the mixture turns golden. Remove from heat. Add the remaining water carefully. Stir well. Spoon the caramel over the pudding.

Put the baking dish (or dishes) on the bottom shelf of the oven and lower the oven to 250° F (120° C). Cook for 2 to 3 hours. The top will be evenly golden when done. Refrigerate until serving time.

Yield: 10 servings.
Each serving contains:
Calories (Kcal): 174
Carbohydrates (g): 32
Sodium (mg): 100

Total fat (g): 2
Protein (g): 7
Cholesterol (mg): 8

Diabetic exchange: 1 skim milk; 1 fruit; ½ fat

Turkish Rice Pudding

Plump the raisins in water before putting them in this pudding.

¼ C	golden raisins	60 mL
	hot water to cover	
2¾ C	lowfat 1% milk	685 mL
½ C	rice	125 mL
½ C	heavy cream	125 mL
2 T	sugar	30 mL
¼ C	dates, pitted and chopped	60 mL
2 t	orange peel, grated	10 mL
½ t	cinnamon	3 mL
4 large	egg yolks or equivalent egg substitute	4 large
¾ t	vanilla extract	4 mL

Put the raisins in a small dish and cover with hot water. Let stand for about half an hour. Drain. Heat 2 cups (500 mL) of the milk in a heavy saucepan and add the rice; stir. Simmer until tender.

Stir in the remaining ¾ cup (185 mL) milk, drained raisins, cream, sugar, dates, orange peel, and cinnamon. Heat again to simmering, stirring occasionally. In a small bowl, beat the egg yolks and vanilla extract together. Remove about a cup of the hot rice mixture and combine it with the egg yolks, then stir this mixture into the pot of rice. Turn into a lightly greased one-quart (1 L) casserole. Bake in a preheated 350° F (180° C) oven for about 25 minutes. The top will be lightly browned.

Yield: 10 servings.
Each serving contains:

Calories (Kcal): 160
Carbohydrates (g): 20
Sodium (mg): 42

Total fat (g): 7
Protein (g): 4
Cholesterol (mg): 42

Diabetic exchange: ½ whole milk; 1 fruit; ½ fat

Italian Rice Pudding Torte

Drier than northern European rice puddings, this is more like a cake. It's delicious with fancy coffee.

4 C	water	1 L
½ C	rice	125 mL
7 large	eggs or equivalent egg substitute	7 large
½ C	sugar	125 mL
¼ C	rum	60 mL
4 t	lemon or lime peel, grated	20 mL
2 T	orange peel, grated	30 mL
2 t	vanilla extract	10 mL
¼ t	salt	2 mL
2 C	lowfat 1% milk	500 mL
2 T	lowfat 1% milk	30 mL

Combine the water and rice in a heavy saucepan and cook over medium heat until boiling. Lower heat and let simmer for 10 minutes. Drain the rice and let it cool. In an electric mixing bowl, beat the eggs well. Add the sugar and continue beating until very pale. Add the rum, lemon or lime peel, orange peel, vanilla extract, and salt. Mix well. Whisk in the 2 C milk.

Butter a 9-inch (23 cm) round baking dish. Spread the rice on the bottom and pour the milk mixture over it. Bake in a preheated 350° F (180° C) oven for about 45 minutes, until the top is a deep golden color.

Yield: 12 servings.
Each serving contains:

Calories (Kcal): 133 — Total fat (g): 3
Carbohydrates (g): 17 — Protein (g): 6
Sodium (mg): 106 — Cholesterol (mg): 126
Diabetic exchange: 1 lowfat milk

Philippine Coconut Rice Pudding

A rice pudding with the sweet surprise of coconut—a true taste of the Pacific.

1 C	rice	250 mL
1¾ C	lowfat 1% milk	435 g
⅓ t	salt	2 mL
2½ C	coconut flakes, packed	625 mL
⅓ t	vanilla extract	2 mL
1 t	coconut extract (optional)	5 mL

Wash the rice several times, cover with water, and soak for one hour. Drain thoroughly and combine in a saucepan with the milk, coconut flakes, and salt. Cover, bring to a boil, and reduce heat to very low. Cook without stirring until the rice is soft. Add the flavorings and serve hot.

Yield: 8 servings.
Each serving contains:

Calories (Kcal): 217   Total fat (g): 8
Carbohydrates (g): 32   Protein (g): 4
Sodium (mg): 176   Cholesterol (mg): 2
Diabetic exchange: 1 starch; 1 fruit; 1½ fat

Mexican Pineapple Rice Pudding

You can make this in an hour while the rest of your dinner is cooking. It's easily made from ingredients on your shelf.

1 can (8 oz.)	crushed pineapple	1 can (227 g)
¼ C	seedless raisins	60 mL
3 C	white rice, raw	750 mL
6 C	water	1500 mL
12 oz.	evaporated milk	340 g
1 t	almond extract	5 mL
2 t	cinnamon	10 mL
½ t	nutmeg	3 mL
	chopped nuts (optional)	

Drain the pineapple, saving the juice in a small bowl. Stir the raisins into the juice. Set aside. In a large saucepan, bring the water to a rolling boil. Stir in the rice and cover the pan. Reduce the heat to very low. Cook for 30 minutes, or until the water is absorbed and the rice is tender. Add the remaining ingredients, except the nuts. Turn into a serving dish. Cool. Garnish with nuts before serving, if desired.

Yield: 12 servings.
Each serving contains:

Calories (Kcal): 229

Total fat (g): 2

Carbohydrates (g): 46

Protein (g): 5

Sodium (mg): 33

Cholesterol (mg): 8

Diabetic exchange: 2 starch; 1 fruit

Danish Rice and Almond Dessert

A traditional Scandinavian Christmas dessert.

1 qt.	lowfat 1% milk	1 L
3 T	sugar	45 mL
¾ C	long-grain rice	185 mL
½ C	almonds, blanched and chopped	125 mL
¼ C	Sherry (or apple juice)	60 mL
2 t	vanilla extract	10 mL

Bring the milk to a boil in a two-quart (2 L) saucepan and add the sugar and rice. Stir once or twice, then lower the heat and simmer uncovered about 25 minutes, or until the rice is soft. Pour into a shallow bowl. Add the chopped almonds, Sherry (or apple juice), and vanilla extract. Cool.

Yield: 10 servings.
Each serving contains:

Calories (Kcal): 142
Carbohydrates (g): 19
Sodium (mg): 52

Total fat (g): 5
Protein (g): 5
Cholesterol (mg): 4

Diabetic exchange: 1 starch, 1 fat

Hawaiian Sweet Potato Pudding

This is really a treat. Even people who aren't sure about sweet potatoes love this. When I'm baking sweet potatoes I bake a few extra and make this pudding the following night. If you're using leftovers, start with the second step.

3 medium	sweet potatoes, peeled	3 medium
2½ C	coconut flakes, packed	625 mL
1½ C	lowfat 1% milk	375 mL

Slice the raw sweet potatoes and boil them until soft. When cooked, mash with a fork or blend in a food processor. Put the mashed sweet potatoes in a saucepan with the coconut flakes and milk. Cook, stirring frequently, until they pudding has the consistency of a thick batter. This pudding may be served hot or cold.

Yield: 8 servings.
Each serving contains:

Calories (Kcal): 180
Carbohydrates (g): 25
Sodium (mg): 89

Total fat (g): 8
Protein (g): 3
Cholesterol (mg): 2

Diabetic exchange: 1 starch; 1 fruit; 1 fat

Chinese Almond Cream

You might like to try 3 T (45 mL) of Amaretto in place of the almond extract in this recipe.

4 C	lowfat 1% milk	1 L
1 C	raw almonds, blanched	250 mL
¼ C	sugar	60 mL
¼ C	rice flour	60 mL
½ t	almond extract	3 mL
1 C	fresh strawberries or other berries	250 mL

Put 3½ cups of the milk in a large saucepan. Add the almonds and sugar. Bring to a boil over a low-to-medium flame, stirring occasionally. Remove from heat, cover, and let stand for 45 minutes. Strain the mixture through a colander set over a bowl. With the back of a wooden spoon press down hard on the almonds. Discard any almonds that don't fit through the holes. Return the liquid to the saucepan. In a small bowl, mix the rice flour with the remaining ½ cup of milk. Pour this into the saucepan and return to low heat. Simmer for about 15 minutes. Stir frequently. The custard should be thick enough to coat the spoon. Add the almond extract and stir. Strain through the colander and spoon into a serving bowl. Cover with plastic wrap and chill for at least two hours. Garnish with berries just before serving.

Yield: 10 servings.
Each serving contains:

Calories (Kcal): 164

Total fat (g): 9

Carbohydrates (g): 16

Protein (g): 7

Sodium (mg): 51

Cholesterol (mg): 4

Diabetic exchange: 1 whole milk

Scottish Crowdie Cream

This is real "Mom" food. You can use 1½ T (25 mL) water and 1 t (5 mL) rum extract instead of rum if you like.

⅓ C	regular oatmeal, uncooked	90 mL
2 C	low-fat frozen non-dairy whipped topping	500 mL
2 T	dark rum	30 mL

Toast the dry oatmeal in a dry frying pan or skillet. When the flakes are a rich golden-brown, quickly remove them from the pan into a bowl to avoid burning. Spoon the whipped topping into a bowl and stir in the rum. Using a rubber spatula, fold in the toasted oatmeal. Put the crowdie cream into custard cups and serve at once.

Yield: 4 servings.
Each serving contains:

Calories (Kcal): 105	Total fat (g): 0
Carbohydrates (g): 12	Protein (g): 1
Sodium (mg): 108	Cholesterol (mg): 0
Diabetic exchange: 1 starch	

German Bavarian Cream

Smooth and luscious, this Bavarian cream melts in your mouth.

1 pkg.	unflavored gelatin	1 pkg.
¼ C	lowfat 1% milk, cold	60 mL
4 large	egg yolks or equivalent egg substitute	4 large
¼ C	sugar	60 mL
1 C	lowfat 1% milk	250 mL
1 t	vanilla extract	5 mL
1 C	low-fat frozen non-dairy whipped topping	250 mL

Put the gelatin in a cup. Stir in the ¼ cup (60 mL) of cold milk. Set it aside. Put the egg yolks in a mixing bowl and beat until thickened. Gradually beat in the sugar. In the top of a double boiler or in a saucepan, heat the cup (250 mL) of milk to scalding. At the same time, heat water in the bottom of a double boiler or large saucepan. Combine the egg mixture with the hot milk and place over boiling water. Cook, stirring constantly, until thick enough to coat a spoon. Remove the mixture from the heat. Using a wire whisk, stir in the vanilla extract and gelatin mixture, stirring until smooth. Refrigerate for about 30 minutes. Fold in the whipped topping. Refrigerate for another two hours until firm. Serve chilled.

Yield: 6 servings.
Each serving contains:

Calories (Kcal): 122	Total fat (g): 4
Carbohydrates (g): 15	Protein (g): 4
Sodium (mg): 47	Cholesterol (mg): 144

Diabetic exchange: 1 starch; ½ fat

Hungarian Fruit Cream

Use any fresh fruit berries in season for this fruit cream.

¾ C	lowfat 1% milk	185 mL
4 T	sugar	60 mL
2 large	egg yolks	2 large
1 env.	gelatin powder, unsweetened	1 env.
2 T	hot water	30 mL
½ C	any fruit purée	125 mL
2 C	low-fat frozen non-dairy whipped topping	500 mL

Boil the milk with half the sugar. In the top of a double boiler over simmering water, whip the eggs yolks and the rest of the sugar. While whipping constantly, add the milk to the egg yolks. Continue stirring until the mixture thickens to a custard. Remove from heat and stir until lukewarm. Add the gelatin and mix well. Add the fruit purée. Fold in the whipped topping. Pour into dessert glasses. Refrigerate and serve chilled.

Yield: 6 servings.
Each serving contains:

Calories (Kcal): 161

Total fat (g): 2

Carbohydrates (g): 17

Protein (g): 14

Sodium (mg): 72

Cholesterol (mg): 72

Diabetic exchange: 1 skim milk; 1 medium-fat meat

Italian Strawberry Ice Cream

This ice cream works very well without an ice cream maker. The more you beat it, the smoother it will be.

3 C	low-fat frozen non-dairy whipped topping	750 mL
1½ C	all-fruit strawberry jam	375 mL

Put the whipped topping into a mixing bowl and let sit at room temperature for about 15 minutes. Gently fold in the puréed strawberry jam. Transfer to shallow trays, such as ice cube trays, and freeze for 1 to 2 hours. Tip the frozen mixture into a bowl. Use a wooden spoon or electric mixer to break up the crystals. Return the mixture to the trays and freeze for another hour or two. Repeat the process again, mixing the ice cream, and freeze for two to three hours before serving.

Yield: 8 servings.
Each serving contains:

Calories (Kcal): 198	Total fat (g): 0
Carbohydrates (g): 42	Protein (g): 0
Sodium (mg): 30	Cholesterol (mg): 0
Diabetic exchange: 3 fruit	

Italian Custard and Berries

Marsala can be replaced by Sherry or a liqueur that you like.

2 T	sugar	30 mL
2 t	cornstarch	10 mL
¾ C	lowfat 1% milk	185 mL
1 large	egg, beaten, or equivalent egg substitute	1 large
¼ C	fat-free sour cream	60 mL
2 T	marsala wine	30 mL
2 C	berries, fresh	500 mL
½ t	cinnamon	3 mL
½ t	ground nutmeg	3 mL

In a heavy saucepan whisk together the sugar and cornstarch. Stir in the milk. Cook over medium heat, stirring frequently until thick and bubbly. Cook for two minutes. Remove from heat. Put the egg into a mixing bowl. Gradually pour about half the hot mixture into the egg, stirring constantly. Return to the saucepan. Cook until nearly boiling, but do not boil. Pour into a serving bowl; stir in the sour cream and marsala. Cover with plastic wrap. Chill the custard for at least two hours before serving. Spoon the berries into dessert dishes. Spoon the custard over the berries. Sprinkle with cinnamon or nutmeg.

Yield: 4 servings.
Each serving contains:
Calories (Kcal): 105
Carbohydrates (g): 17
Sodium (mg): 53
Diabetic exchange: 1 starch

Total fat (g): 2
Protein (g): 4
Cholesterol (mg): 56

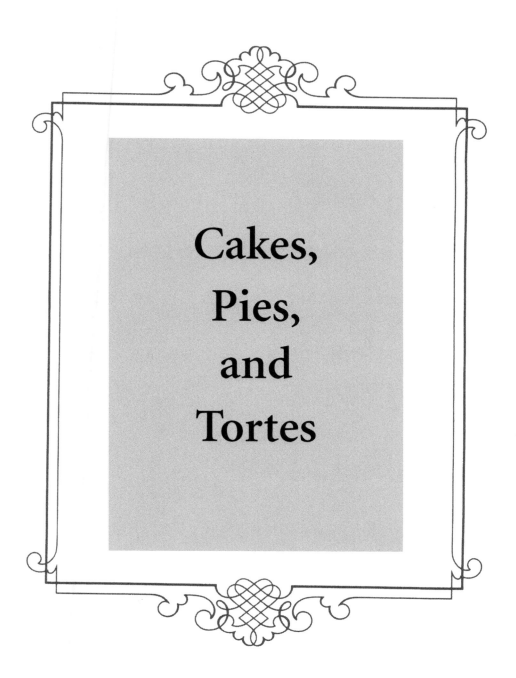

Cakes,
Pies,
and
Tortes

Irish Jam Cake

All-fruit jams and jellies usually need to be diluted with a little water to become spreadable. As an optional garnish, fresh berries are lovely. This is a light and lovely cake.

1¾ C	cake flour, sifted	435 mL
¾ t	baking powder	185 mL
⅛ t	salt	1 mL
4 large	eggs or equivalent egg substitute, room temperature	4 large
½ C	granulated sugar	125 mL
1 t	lemon rind, grated	5 mL
¾ C	lemon extract	185 mL
½ C	all-fruit blueberry jam, and water to dilute	125 mL

Stir together the flour, baking powder, and salt in a small bowl and set aside. Grease and flour two 8-inch (20 cm) cake pans and line the bottom of each with an 8-inch round parchment or waxed paper circle. In a large mixing bowl beat the eggs until they are thick and lemon-colored. Gradually beat in the sugar. Using a spatula, fold in the flour mixture, lemon rind, and lemon extract. Spread in cake pans. Bake in a 350° F (180° C) oven for 20 to 25 minutes, or until a toothpick inserted in the center comes out clean. Cool slightly before turning out onto a cooling rack and remove the waxed paper immediately. Cool completely before putting one layer on a serving plate. Add a small amount of water to the jam and mix with a fork to make this jam soft enough to spread. Spread the jam on the first layer and top with the second layer.

Yield: 12 servings.
Each serving contains:
Calories (Kcal): 164   Total fat (g): 2
Carbohydrates (g): 29   Protein (g): 4
Sodium (mg): 66   Cholesterol (mg): 71
Diabetic exchange: 1 starch; 1 fruit

Spanish Marmalade Pudding

Although this is called a pudding, it's more like a loaf cake with orange frosting.

1 C	all-purpose flour	250 mL
1½ t	baking powder	8 mL
½ t	ground cinnamon	3 mL
¼ t	salt	2 mL
4 T	butter, margarine, or fat-free butter and oil replacement	60 mL
⅓ C	sugar	80 mL
3 large	eggs or equivalent egg substitute, lightly beaten	3 large
½ C	lowfat 1% milk	125 mL
1 t	orange peel, grated fine	5 mL
1 t	vanilla extract	5 mL
1 C	all-fruit marmalade jam	250 mL

In a large bowl, sift the flour, baking powder, cinnamon, and salt. In another large bowl, cream the butter and sugar until light and fluffy. Beat in the eggs. Beat in the flour mixture, ¼ cup (60 mL) at a time, alternating with the milk. Beat in the orange peel and vanilla extract.

Melt the marmalade in a small pan over low heat. Stir constantly. Pour the marmalade into a well-greased 9 × 5 × 3-inch (23 × 12 × 8 cm) loaf pan. Spoon in the batter. Bake in a preheated 350° F (180° C) oven for 40 to 50 minutes. A cake tester inserted in the center will come out clean.

Cool in the pan for about 10 minutes. Run a knife around the edges of the pan. Invert onto a serving plate. Slice and serve warm.

Yield: 10 servings.
Each serving contains:

Calories (Kcal): 220	Total fat (g): 6
Carbohydrates (g): 36	Protein (g): 4
Sodium (mg): 179	Cholesterol (mg): 77

Diabetic exchange: 1 starch; 1 fat; 1 fruit

Italian Pear Crisp

The European taste comes from boiling spices in the wine.

½ C	raisins	125 mL
1½ C	red wine	375 mL
⅓ C	sugar	80 mL
1 t	cinnamon	5 mL
2 whole	cloves	2 whole
1 t	orange extract	5 mL
2 strips	orange peel (about ⅛ of a medium orange)	2 strips
2 cans (16 oz.)	pears, packed in juice	2 cans (900 g)
3 C	whole wheat bread crumbs	750 mL
3 T	butter	45 mL
6 T	frozen non-dairy whipped topping (optional)	90 mL

Put the raisins in a small bowl. Cover with hot water and set aside. In a medium-size enamel saucepan, bring to a boil the red wine, sugar, cinnamon, cloves, orange extract, and lemon peel. Gently boil for 30 minutes, until slightly concentrated. Drain the pears and slice them into bite-size pieces. Add them to the wine and boil for five minutes more. Drain the pears and raisins, discard the cloves and lemon peel, and reserve the cooking liquid.

Butter a one-quart (1 L) glass baking dish and cover the bottom with one cup (250 mL) of the bread crumbs. On top of the layer of crumbs arrange one third of the poached pear slices and several raisins. Continue layering until you have used all the ingredients, finishing with bread crumbs. Pour the reserved cooking liquid over the top and dot with butter.

Bake in a preheated 350° F (180° C) oven for 45 minutes. Serve warm with frozen non-dairy whipped topping, if desired.

Yield: 12 servings.
Each serving contains:

Calories (Kcal): 242	Total fat (g): 5
Carbohydrates (g): 43	Protein (g): 4
Sodium (mg): 220	Cholesterol (mg): 8

Diabetic exchange: 1 starch; 2 fruit; 1 fat

Swiss Pear Tart

The first time I made this, I left it cooling and went out to run an errand. When I came home, serious inroads had been made in tart consumption! Everyone loved it.

1 whole	prepared pie crust	1 whole
1¼ C	applesauce, unsweetened	310 mL
13 oz.	pear halves in juice, sliced, drained	370 g
⅓ C	sugar	80 mL
1 C	dry red wine	250 mL
3 T (approx.)	juice of half a lemon	45 mL
1 pinch	cinnamon	1 pinch
1 pinch	ground cloves	1 pinch
2 T	cornstarch	30 mL
2 T	water	30 mL
2 T	all-fruit raspberry jam	30 mL
8 T	low-fat frozen non-dairy whipped topping (optional)	120 mL

In a blender or food processor, purée the applesauce and one half the drained pear halves. Pour the mixture into a saucepan and add the sugar, wine, lemon juice, cinnamon, and cloves. In a teacup, blend the cornstarch and water together until the cornstarch dissolves. Add the cornstarch to the applesauce and mix well. Cook at just below boiling, stirring frequently, until reduced to a thick purée. Cool. Pour the purée into the prepared pie crust and bake in a preheated 425° F (220° C) oven for 30 minutes. Remove from the oven, and arrange the remaining pear slices on top of the purée. Bake for 10 more minutes. Remove to a cooling rack. When slightly cooled, spread the top with jam. Refrigerate until ready to serve. Top with whipped topping, if desired.

Yield: 8 servings.
Each serving contains:

Calories (Kcal): 117	Total fat (g): 0
Carbohydrates (g): 25	Protein (g): 0
Sodium (mg): 5	Cholesterol (mg): 0
Diabetic exchange: 2 fruit	

Israeli Passover Sponge Cake

The trick to keeping this cake from falling is to have a long-necked bottle—a wine or soda bottle—ready to invert the cake onto so it cools upside down.

5	egg whites	5
2 T	sugar	30 mL
5 large	egg yolks	5 large
1 whole	orange peel, grated	1 whole
1 whole	lemon peel, grated	1 whole
¼ C	orange juice	60 mL
2 T	lemon juice	30 mL
¾ C	matzo meal	185 mL
½ C	potato flour or cornstarch (see note)	125 mL
2 T	sugar	30 mL
½ t	salt	3 mL
½ C	vegetable oil	125 mL

Beat egg whites until foamy. Gradually add the sugar and beat until stiff peaks form. Set aside. In another bowl mix the yolks well and add the lemon and orange peels and juice. In another bowl, sift together the matzo meal, potato flour, 2 T (30 mL) sugar, and salt. Stir. Make a well in the center and pour in the yolk-juice mixture and the oil. Beat well. Carefully fold the egg whites into the egg yolk mixture. Keep in as much air as possible so the cake will be light. Spoon the batter into an ungreased tube pan. Bake in the center of a preheated 350° F (175° C) oven for 50 to 60 minutes or until a tester comes out clean. When the cake is done, take it out of the oven and immediately invert over the neck of a bottle, so it hangs upside down to cool. When the cake has cooled completely, gently remove it from the tube pan with a knife.

Note: Many kosher cooks do not use cornstarch on Passover.

Yield: 20 servings.
Each serving contains:

Calories (Kcal): 94	Total fat (g): 7
Carbohydrates (g): 7	Protein (g): 2
Sodium (mg): 70	Cholesterol (mg): 53

Diabetic exchange: ½ starch; 1 fat

Chinese Steamed Sponge Cake

You can steam this cake in a bamboo steamer or on the metal tray of an electric wok. Watch the water level so it doesn't run dry.

5 large	eggs, or equivalent egg substitute, at room temperature	5 large
1 T	water	15 mL
½ C	sugar	125 mL
1 C	cake flour	250 mL
1 T	butter, margarine, or fat-free replacement, melted	15 mL

Put the eggs, water, and sugar in a mixing bowl and beat for 10 minutes at high speed. The mixture will become thick and creamy. Fold in the flour, then the melted butter. Line the bottom of a 9-inch (23 cm) round baking pan with parchment paper. Pour the batter into the pan. Heat the water in a wok to boiling. Set the cake pan on the steaming rack and cover. Steam 20 minutes at medium heat. A toothpick inserted in the center will come out clean when done. Turn the cake out and peel off the paper. Serve warm or cold.

Yield: 12 servings.
Each serving contains:

Calories (Kcal): 104

Carbohydrates (g): 16

Sodium (mg): 36

Diabetic exchange: 1 starch

Total fat (g): 3

Protein (g): 3

Cholesterol (mg): 91

Polish Baked Cheese Pastry

If they don't think they like cottage cheese, they'll never know it's in this dish.

6 whole	eggs, separated	6 whole
4 T	unsalted butter	60 mL
½ C	cottage cheese	125 mL
⅓ C	sugar	90 mL
½ C	almonds, chopped fine (optional)	125 mL
3 T	bread crumbs	45 mL
1 t	bread crumbs	5 mL

Cream the egg yolks and butter. Add the cottage cheese and sugar and continue mixing until smooth. Add the almonds and mix thoroughly. Beat egg whites. Add the 3 T (45 mL) bread crumbs to the egg whites a little at a time. Grease an 8- or 9-inch (20–23 cm) cake pan generously. Coat with 1 teaspoon (5 mL) bread crumbs. Fold the egg whites and bread crumbs into the cottage cheese mixture. Pour the batter into the prepared pan. Bake in a preheated 350° F (180° C) oven for 30 minutes.

Yield: 8 servings.
Each serving contains:
Calories (Kcal): 166   Total fat (g): 10
Carbohydrates (g): 11   Protein (g): 7
Sodium (mg): 125   Cholesterol (mg): 177
Diabetic exchange: 1 whole milk

Italian Cheesecake

This is a flavorful and traditional Italian cheesecake. It's not like "New York" cheesecake. When I serve this I don't tell people it's cheesecake, and they love it.

Pastry

1½ C	all-purpose flour	375 mL
¼ C	unsalted butter, chilled and cut into bits	60 mL
¼ C	fat-free cream cheese	60 mL
2 T	sugar	30 mL
2 large	egg yolks	2 large
1 t	lemon peel, grated	5 mL
1 T	dry marsala wine	15 mL

Filling

3 T	almonds, toasted (or ground pine nuts)	45 mL
¼ C	golden raisins	60 mL
⅓ C	marsala wine	80 mL
½ lb.	ricotta cheese, part skim milk	225 g
½ lb.	fat-free cream cheese	450 g
¼ C	sugar	60 mL
1 T	all-purpose flour	15 mL
4 large	eggs, separated	4 large
½ C	fat-free sour cream	125 mL
1 t	vanilla extract	5 mL
½ t	lemon extract	3 mL
2 large	egg whites	2 large

In a mixing bowl, mix the flour, butter, and cream cheese until the mixture resembles coarse cornmeal. In another bowl mix the sugar, egg yolks, lemon peel, and marsala and add it to the flour mixture to make a soft dough. Press a thin layer of dough over the bottom and sides of a 9-inch (23 cm) springform pan. Refrigerate at least one hour.

Plump the raisins by putting them in a small saucepan and covering with the marsala. Heat over low heat until warm. Remove from the heat and let stand half an hour.

With an electric mixer, beat the ricotta and cream cheese until fluffy. Add the sugar and flour and beat until blended. Beat in the egg yolks, sour cream, vanilla extract, and lemon extract until fluffy. In a second mixing bowl, beat the 6 egg whites until soft peaks form. Fold in the whites and almonds or pine nuts with the raisins.

Pour the filling into the refrigerated tart shell. Bake in a preheated 350° F (180° C) oven until the filling shimmers but is no longer liquid when jiggled, about 50 to 60 minutes. Cool in the pan for 20 to 30 minutes. Remove the sides of the pan and serve warm.

Yield: 12 servings.
Each serving contains:

Calories (Kcal): 219	Total fat (g): 9
Carbohydrates (g): 24	Protein (g): 8
Sodium (mg): 117	Cholesterol (mg): 124

Diabetic exchange: 1 whole milk; 1 fruit

Israeli Orange-Flavored Cheesecake

A moist and heavy cheesecake with a graham cracker crust, this cheesecake comes from many countries.

Crust

1½ C	graham cracker crumbs	375 mL
2 T	sugar	30 mL
2 T	fat-free cream cheese	30 mL

Filling

1½ lbs.	fat-free cream cheese	675 g
½ C	sugar	125 mL
1 medium	orange rind, finely grated	1 medium
4 large	eggs, separated	4 large
2 T	all-purpose flour	30 mL
⅛ t	salt	1 mL
1 t	vanilla extract	5 mL
½ t	almond extract	3 mL

Blend together the crust ingredients. Press against the bottom and sides of a well-greased 10-inch (25 cm) springform pan. Set aside. Put the cream cheese for the filling in a mixing bowl. Beat until smooth. Set aside. Add the sugar and rind. Beat in the remaining ingredients, except the egg whites, until perfectly smooth. Beat the egg whites until moist peaks form. Fold the egg whites into the cheese mixture. Spoon the filling into the crust.

Bake in a preheated 325° F (165° C) oven for 1½ hours, or until the cake is very firm. Turn off the heat and allow the cake to remain in the oven for an additional 30 minutes. The cake will sink as it cools. Remove from the oven and cool to room temperature in the pan. Carefully remove the springform. Refrigerate the cheesecake for a minimum of three hours. For best results, refrigerate overnight.

Yield: 12 servings.
Each serving contains:

Calories (Kcal): 209	Total fat (g): 8
Carbohydrates (g): 40	Protein (g): 7
Sodium (mg): 326	Cholesterol (mg): 94

Diabetic exchange: 1 whole milk; 1 fruit

Polish Cheesecake

A very light and fluffy cheesecake with the authentic cheesecake taste you want.

⅔ C	zwieback crumbs, packed	180 mL
18 oz.	fat-free cream cheese, softened	500 g
½ C	fat-free sour cream	125 mL
1 t	vanilla extract	5 mL
5 whole	egg whites	5 whole
⅓ C	granulated sugar	90 mL

Sprinkle the bottom and sides of a buttered 8-inch (20 cm) springform pan with zwieback crumbs, pressing any extra crumbs evenly on the bottom of the pan. Put the cream cheese into a mixing bowl. Add the sour cream and vanilla extract and mix until fluffy. In another bowl beat the egg whites until foamy. Beat in sugar to egg whites gradually, beating well after each addition. Beat until whites are stiff enough to hold a peak but not dry. Fold gently into the cheese mixture. Turn the mixture into the springform pan lined with zwieback. Bake in a preheated 350° (180° C) pan for 25 minutes. Remove from the oven (the center will still be soft); let cool away from drafts. When cooled, refrigerate for four hours. Remove the outside of the springform pan. Cut the cake into serving pieces and garnish with fruit as desired.

Yield: 12 servings.
Each serving contains:

Calories (Kcal): 129	Total fat (g): 1
Carbohydrates (g): 16	Protein (g): 6
Sodium (mg): 188	Cholesterol (mg): 11

Diabetic exchange: 1 starch; ½ lean meat

Eastern European Fresh Apple Cake

Many countries have a recipe for apple cake similar to this one with very minor flavor variations. It's a great fall or winter dessert. This is a moist cake and the apple glaze is subtle.

¼ C	butter, margarine, or fat-free butter and oil replacement	60 mL
¼ C	fat-free cream cheese	60 mL
¼ C	brown sugar	60 mL
¼ C	granulated sugar	60 mL
1 large	egg	1 large
1½ C	flour, sifted	375 mL
½ t	baking soda	3 mL
½ t	baking powder	3 mL
½ t	salt	3 mL
½ t	cinnamon	3 mL
¼ t	nutmeg	2 mL
⅛ t	ground cloves	1 mL
½ C	buttermilk (see note)	125 mL
1½ C	fresh raw apples, diced	375 mL

Topping

1 T	brown sugar	15 mL
½ t	cinnamon	3 mL
¼ C	chopped walnuts (optional)	60 mL

Note: Substitute ½ cup (125 mL) milk and 2 T (30 mL) vinegar for the buttermilk, if desired.

In a mixing bowl, cream the butter, cream cheese, and sugars. Add egg and beat well. In another bowl, sift the flour with baking powder, baking soda, salt, and spices. Add to creamed mixture alternately with the buttermilk. Fold in the apples. Turn into a well-greased 9-inch (23 cm) square baking pan. Mix together topping and sprinkle on top. Bake in a preheated 350° F (180° C) oven for 40 minutes or until the cake springs back when touched.

Yield: 12 servings.
Each serving contains:
Calories (Kcal): 144
Carbohydrates (g): 23
Sodium (mg): 190
Total fat (g): 5
Protein (g): 3
Cholesterol (mg): 29
Diabetic exchange: 1 starch; 1 fat

German Apple Kuchen

German apple cake needs just one apple; the flavor comes from shredding the apple.

1½ C	flour, sifted	375 mL
¼ C	sugar	60 mL
2 t	baking powder	10 mL
½ t	salt	3 mL
½ t	cinnamon	3 mL
½ C	walnuts, chopped	125 mL
1 whole	apple, peeled and shredded	1 whole
1 large	egg or equivalent egg substitute, lightly beaten	1 large
½ C	lowfat 1% milk	125 mL
3 T	canola oil	45 mL
½ C	fat-free sour cream	125 mL
¼ C	sugar	60 mL

Sift together the flour, sugar, baking powder, salt, and cinnamon into a large mixing bowl. Remove 2 T (30 mL) walnuts and set them aside. Mix the remaining nuts and shredded apple into the flour mixture. In another bowl, mix together the egg, milk, and oil. Pour this onto the flour mixture and stir until well mixed. Turn into a well-greased 9-inch (23 cm) cake pan. Spoon the sour cream onto the top. Sprinkle with the remaining ¼ cup (60 mL) of sugar and top with the walnuts. Bake in a preheated 400° F (200° F) oven for 30–35 minutes. Serve warm.

Yield: 12 servings.
Each serving contains:

Calories (Kcal): 175

Carbohydrates (g): 24

Sodium (mg): 168

Diabetic exchange: 2 starch

Total fat (g): 7

Protein (g): 4

Cholesterol (mg): 19

German Apple Strudel

Apple strudel oozes good feelings and a hearty welcome. Your family and guests will be very impressed.

Dough

2 C	flour	500 mL
1 large	egg or equivalent egg substitute, lightly beaten	1 large
1 T	canola oil	15 mL
½ t	salt	3 mL
⅔ C	warm water	165 mL

Filling

4 T	butter, margarine, or fat-free butter and oil replacement	60 mL
½ C	dry bread crumbs	125 mL
4 large	apples, peeled, cored, and sliced	4 large
¼ C	sugar	60 mL
1 T	cinnamon	15 mL
½ C	raisins	125 mL

Glaze frosting

1 large	egg yolk	1 large
1 t	sugar	5 mL
1 T	water	15 mL

Put the flour in a mixing bowl. In another bowl mix together the egg, oil, salt, and warm water. Pour the liquid onto the flour and mix thoroughly. Turn out onto a well-floured work surface. Knead the dough until it is smooth and elastic. Cover with a tea towel or plastic wrap and let sit for 15 minutes.

Meanwhile, make the filling by melting the butter in a saucepan. Add the bread crumbs and brown just until golden. Roll out the dough on a well-floured work surface. Make it as thin as possible. Sprinkle the bread crumbs evenly over the surface of the dough. In a mixing bowl coat the apple slices with the sugar and cinnamon by tossing lightly. Add the raisins and mix again. Spread this mixture evenly on top of the bread crumbs. Roll the long way. Seal the dough together with your fingers. Mix the egg yolk, sugar, and water together and brush the top of the roll. Sprinkle the top with the sugar. Bake in a preheated 400° F (200° C) oven for 30–35 minutes. Serve hot or cold.

Yield: 16 slices.
Each serving contains:

Calories (Kcal): 159

Total fat (g): 5

Carbohydrates (g): 27

Protein (g): 3

Sodium (mg): 125

Cholesterol (mg): 27

Diabetic exchange: 1 starch; ½ fruit; 1 fat

Italian Apple Cake

Using firm cooking apples will keep distinct apple segments in the cake. Softer apples will disappear in the baking, but the cake will still be rich and great.

2 large	egg yolks	2 large
⅓ C	flour	(80 mL)
1 T	sugar	15 mL
1 pinch	salt	1 pinch
¼ C	lowfat 1% milk	60 mL
2 lbs.	apples, peeled and sliced	900 g
2 large	egg whites, beaten until stiff	2 large

In a mixing bowl, beat the egg yolks until well mixed. Add the flour, sugar, salt, and milk. Mix well. Add the apples and mix. Fold in the beaten egg whites. Pour the mixture into a buttered 10-inch (25 cm) cake pan. Bake in a preheated 350° F (180° C) oven for about 45 minutes. A cake tester inserted in the center will come out dry. Cool on a wire rack.

Yield: 8 servings.
Each serving contains:

Calories (Kcal): 114	Total fat (g): 12
Carbohydrates (g): 23	Protein (g): 3
Sodium (mg): 36	Cholesterol (mg): 53

Diabetic exchange: 1 starch; 1 fruit

Italian Apple Tart

Made like a cheesecake in a springform pan, this tart is very elegant.

Pastry

1½ C	all-purpose flour	375 mL
¼ C	unsalted butter, chilled and cut into bits	60 mL
¼ C	fat-free cream cheese	60 mL
2 T	sugar	30 mL
2 large	egg yolks	2 large
1 t	lemon peel, grated	5 mL
1 T	dry marsala wine	15 mL

Filling

5 whole	apples—peeled, cored, and cut into 8 pieces	5 whole
¼ C	honey	60 mL
1 whole	grated lemon peel	1 whole
½ whole	grated orange peel	½ whole
½ whole	juice of orange	½ whole
1 whole	juice of lemon	1 whole
¼ C	Grand Marnier liqueur	60 mL

In a mixing bowl mix the flour, butter, and cream cheese until the mixture resembles coarse cornmeal. In another bowl mix the sugar, egg yolks, lemon peel, and marsala and add to the flour mixture, making a soft dough. Press a thin layer of dough over the bottom and sides of a 9-inch (23 cm) springform pan.

Bake in a preheated 375° F (200° C) oven for 10 minutes. Cool on a wire rack and then refrigerate. Put all the remaining ingredients in a frying pan. Stir well. Turn the heat on and cook, stirring frequently until the apples are cooked just to the point of tenderness. They should be dry. Cool.

Pour the filling into the refrigerated pie shell. Bake in a preheated 350° F (180° C) oven until the filling shimmers but is no longer liquid when jiggled, 50–60 minutes. Let cool in the pan 20–30 minutes. Remove the side of the pan and serve warm.

Yield: 8 servings.
Each serving contains:

Calories (Kcal): 185	Total fat (g): 8
Carbohydrates (g): 26	Protein (g): 3
Sodium (mg): 147	Cholesterol (mg): 27

Diabetic exchange: 1 starch; 1 fruit; 1 fat

German Poppy Seed Cake

This cake calls for a lot of poppy seeds, so buy them in bulk.

2 C	poppy seeds, dried	500 mL
6 C	water	1.5 L
¼ C	butter, margarine, or fat-free butter and oil replacement	60 mL
¼ C	fat-free cream cheese	60 mL
1 T	fat-free sour cream	15 mL
⅓ C	sugar	80 mL
1 C	flour	250 mL
2 t	baking powder	10 mL
7 large	egg whites	7 large
½ t	anise or licorice flavoring	3 mL

Put the poppy seeds in a bowl, cover with boiling water, and stir until they are soaked. Cool. Cover with plastic wrap and let stand overnight. Carefully drain the poppy seeds in a fine colander lined with a tea towel or fine mesh strainer. Discard the soaking liquid. Spoon the seeds into a food processor or blender and grind well.

In a large mixing bowl, beat the butter, cream cheese, and sour cream together until well mixed and creamy. Beat in the sugar. In a small bowl combine the flour and baking powder. Beat the dry ingredients into the butter and sugar mixture. Beat in the ground poppy seeds. In a large mixing bowl, beat the egg whites until stiff. Add the anise or other flavoring to the egg whites and beat well. Fold the flavored egg whites into the butter and flour mixture. Spoon the batter into a well-greased and floured 10-inch (25 cm) springform pan and bake in a preheated 350° F (180° C) oven for one hour. A cake tester will come out clean. Cool on a wire rack for a few minutes before removing the sides. Let the cake cool completely before cutting.

Yield: 14 servings.
Each serving contains:

Calories (Kcal): 200	Total fat (g): 12
Carbohydrates (g): 17	Protein (g): 8
Sodium (mg): 133	Cholesterol (mg): 10

Diabetic exchange: 1 starch; 1 medium-fat meat; 1 fat

Polish Easter Cake

This is a yeast cake, so it needs time to rise. It's a perfect cake to make when you're home all day.

½ C	lowfat 1% milk	125 mL
¼ C	granulated sugar	60 mL
½ t	salt	3 mL
2 T	butter, margarine, or fat-free butter and oil replacement	30 mL
¼ C	warm water	60 mL
1 env.	yeast	1 env.
2 large	eggs or equivalent egg substitute	2 large
2½ C	all-purpose flour	625 mL
½ C	chopped almonds	125 mL
½ C	raisins	125 mL
½ t	lemon peel	3 mL

Scald the milk in a heavy saucepan. Stir in the sugar, salt, and butter replacement. Set aside to cool. Pour the warm water into a large bowl. Sprinkle yeast over the water; stir until dissolved. Add milk mixture, eggs, and flour and beat vigorously for five minutes. Cover with a tea towel or plastic wrap. Let rise in a warm place, free from draft, for 1½ hours or until doubled in bulk. Stir the batter down and beat in almonds, raisins, and lemon peel. Pour the batter into a greased and floured 1½-quart (1½ L) casserole. Let rise for 1 hour. Bake in a preheated 350° F (180° C) oven 50 minutes. Let cool in pan on a cooling rack for 20 minutes before removing.

Yield: 12 servings.
Each serving contains:

Calories (Kcal): 200
Carbohydrates (g): 31
Sodium (mg): 126

Total fat (g): 6
Protein (g): 6
Cholesterol (mg): 41

Diabetic exchange: 2 starch; 1 fat

Greek New Year's Day Cake

This beautiful cake is served on New Year's Day in Greece with a coin inside. The person who gets the coin in a slice will have the best luck in the new year. The cake is festive any day.

3½ C	all-purpose flour	875 mL
2 t	baking powder	10 mL
½ C	unsalted butter	125 mL
½ C	fat-free cream cheese	125 mL
½ C	sugar	125 mL
2 large	eggs or equivalent egg substitute	2 large
1 large	egg yolk	1 large
1 whole	orange rind, grated	1 whole
¼ t	nutmeg (optional)	2 mL
¼ C	fat-free sour cream	60 mL
1 T	cognac	15 mL
1	silver coin, boiled and wrapped in foil	1
20 whole	almonds, blanched	20 whole
1 large	egg white, beaten until frothy	1 large

Sift the flour and baking powder into a small bowl. In a mixing bowl, beat the butter and cream cheese until fluffy. Gradually add the sugar and beat for four minutes. Add the eggs, one at a time, and then the yolk, beating after each addition. Add the orange rind and nutmeg (if desired.) In another small bowl, combine the sour cream and cognac. Beat this combination into the batter. Add the sifted dry ingredients. Mix in well. Stir in the coin. Spoon batter into a well-greased 10-inch (25 cm) round cake pan, pressing the edge with the tines of a fork to decorate. Arrange the blanched almonds in a decorative pattern on top. Bake in a preheated 350° F (180° C) oven for 15 to 20 minutes, until a cake tester inserted in the center comes out clean. Pull out from the oven, brush with egg white, and return to the oven. Continue baking another 20 minutes. Cool before serving.

Yield: 16 servings.
Each serving contains:

Calories (Kcal): 229

Total fat (g): 10

Carbohydrates (g): 29

Protein (g): 6

Sodium (mg): 83

Cholesterol (mg): 58

Diabetic exchange: 2 starch; 2 fat

Danish Birthday Cake

In Denmark it's traditional to celebrate birthdays at breakfast time. This cake would be made the day before.

3 envs.	yeast	3 envs.
¼ C	warm water	60 mL
⅓ C	sugar	80 mL
3 C	cake flour	750 mL
½ C	lowfat 1% milk	125 mL
2 large	eggs, or equivalent egg substitute, beaten	2 large
⅓ C	butter, margarine, or fat-free replacement, softened	80 mL
½ C	almonds, chopped	125 mL
1 T	lemon peel, grated	15 mL
1 large	egg or equivalent egg substitute, lightly beaten	1 large
1 T	lowfat 1% milk	15 mL
1 T	sugar	15 mL

Dissolve the yeast in the warm water. Sift the sugar with flour and mix in the milk, yeast, and beaten eggs. Turn onto a floured work surface. Knead the dough thoroughly. Turn into an oiled bowl. Cover with plastic wrap or a tea towel and set in a warm place. Let the dough rise until doubled in bulk. This may take an hour or two.

Roll the dough into a rectangle about 6 × 12 inches (15 × 30 cm). Spread the softened butter on the surface. Sprinkle with the nuts and lemon peel. Fold each side of the dough toward the middle and shape the roll into a circle or wreath. Place on a well-greased baking sheet. Cover with a tea towel or plastic wrap and let rise again for an hour in a warm place.

Mix together the egg and milk. Brush the surface of the cake and sprinkle with the sugar. Bake in a preheated 350° F (180° C) oven for 45 to 50 minutes.

Yield: 20 servings.
Each serving contains:

Calories (Kcal): 141	Total fat (g): 6
Carbohydrates (g): 19	Protein (g): 4
Sodium (mg): 46	Cholesterol (mg): 40

Diabetic exchange: 1 starch; 1 fat

Norwegian Cake

A layer cake that's fancy enough for a special occasion.

½ C	butter, margarine, or fat-free replacement	125 mL
½ C	fat-free cream cheese	125 mL
⅓ C	sugar	80 mL
4 large	eggs, separated	4 large
¾ C	flour	185 mL
3 t	baking powder	15 mL
5 T	lowfat 1% milk	75 mL
2 T	powdered sugar	30 mL
2 C	low-fat frozen non-dairy whipped topping	500 mL

In a large mixing bowl, cream together the butter, cream cheese, and sugar. Add the egg yolks and mix well. In another bowl, sift together the flour and baking powder. Add the butter mixture to the flour a little at a time, alternating with the milk. Pour the batter equally into two well-greased 8-inch (20 cm) cake pans. Set aside.

In another mixing bowl, beat the egg whites until foamy. Add the powdered sugar and continue beating until stiff peaks form. Divide the beaten egg whites between the two pans. Bake in a preheated 350° F (180° C) oven for 40 minutes. Cool on wire racks. Just before serving, turn out one pan onto a serving dish and flip so the egg white side is up. Spread half the whipped topping on top of the layer. Put on the second layer and top with the rest of the whipped topping.

Yield: 12 servings.
Each serving contains:

Calories (Kcal): 179	Total fat (g): 9
Carbohydrates (g): 17	Protein (g): 4
Sodium (mg): 234	Cholesterol (mg): 93

Diabetic exchange: 1 starch; 2 fat

German Cake

This cake is very rich and moist, and it's easy to make.

2 T	fat-free sour cream	30 mL
¼ C	fat-free cream cheese	60 mL
½ C	butter, margarine, or fat-free butter and oil replacement	125 mL
¼ C	sugar	60 mL
4 large	eggs, or equivalent egg substitute, at room temperature	4 large
1 T	lemon juice	15 mL
½ T	lemon peel, grated	8 mL
1 C	all-purpose flour	250 mL
1 t	baking powder	5 mL
¼ C	chopped almonds, pecans, or hazelnuts (optional)	60 mL
¼ t	ground cinnamon	2 mL
1 T	sugar	15 mL

Beat the sour cream, cream cheese, and butter in a large bowl. Beat in the sugar and continue mixing until light and creamy. Beat in the eggs, one at a time. Add lemon juice and lemon peel. Beat well. Add the flour and baking powder and beat well to make the batter really smooth. Prepare an 8-inch (20 cm) round baking pan by greasing it well and dusting with flour. Pour the batter into the pan.

In a small dish, mix the nuts (if you're using them) with the cinnamon and sugar. Sprinkle evenly over the top of the batter. Bake in a preheated 350° F (175° C) oven for 30–35 minutes. Cool slightly, and carefully turn out onto a wire rack. Serve warm or at room temperature.

Yield: 12 servings.
Each serving contains:

Calories (Kcal): 156   Total fat (g): 9
Carbohydrates (g): 14   Protein (g): 4
Sodium (mg): 145   Cholesterol (mg): 92
Diabetic exchange: 1 starch; 2 fat

Brazilian Pieces of Love

It's only fitting that this recipe comes from Cristina Junqueira, a lovely friend and colleague.

1 can (20 oz.)	crushed pineapple in water	1 can (567 g)
8 oz.	coconut flakes	240 g
3 large	eggs or equivalent egg substitute	225 g
3 C	flour	750 mL
½ C	sugar	125 mL
1 T	baking soda	15 mL
1 T	butter	15 mL
3 large	eggs or equivalent egg substitute	3 large
2 C	lowfat 1% milk	500 mL

Make the filling first. In a saucepan, combine the pineapple and coconut flakes, including the "water" from the pineapple. Bring to a boil over medium heat and turn the heat to low. Stirring frequently, cook until the water has been absorbed—a cottage cheese consistency. Set aside to cool.

Make the cake by putting the flour into a mixing bowl. Mix in the sugar and baking soda until well combined. In another bowl, beat the butter until soft. Gradually add the eggs. Spoon in the dry mixture and beat until the batter is well combined. Pour half the batter into a well-greased 8 × 11-inch (28 × 27 cm) pan. Spoon the filling carefully over the batter, spreading well. Spoon the remainder of the batter on top. Bake in a preheated 375° F (190° C) oven for 30–35 minutes. The top will be golden brown. Cool on a wire rack before cutting.

Yield: 40 squares.
Each serving contains:

Calories (Kcal): 94	Total fat (g): 3
Carbohydrates (g): 14	Protein (g): 3
Sodium (mg): 128	Cholesterol (mg): 33
Diabetic exchange: 1 starch	

German Almond Torte

Expect raves—this is a very light European torte.

½ C	dry bread crumbs, ground fine	125 mL
½ C	lowfat 1% milk	125 mL
1 t	rum extract, or 1 T rum	5 mL
5 T	butter, margarine, or fat-free butter and oil replacement	75 mL
⅓ C	sugar	80 mL
6 large	egg yolks	6 large
6 large	egg whites, beaten stiffly	6 large
¾ C	ground almonds, toasted lightly in a pan	185 mL
3 C	low-fat frozen non-dairy whipped topping	750 mL
1 t	almond extract	5 mL
2 T	ground almonds	30 mL

In a small bowl, mix together the bread crumbs, milk, and rum flavoring. Set aside. In a larger mixing bowl, beat together the butter and sugar. Add the egg yolks and beat well. Add the soaked crumbs. Beat again. Fold in the egg whites and almonds. Divide into three 8-inch (20 cm) well-greased cake pans. Bake in a preheated 350° F (180° C) oven for 35 minutes. Cool on wire rack. Turn out of tins. Place one cake on a serving plate. Using a whisk, blend the almond extract into the whipped topping. Spread one-third over the cake. Put on the next layer and top with whipped topping. Continue, ending with whipped topping on top. Sprinkle with the remaining almonds.

Yield: 12 servings.
Each serving contains:

Calories (Kcal): 217	Total fat (g): 13
Carbohydrates (g): 16	Protein (g): 6
Sodium (mg): 137	Cholesterol (mg): 120

Diabetic exchange: 1 whole milk; 1 fat

German Meringue Torte

You can use other berries in place of strawberries or even other non-berry fresh fruit. In European baking it's common to see piles of meringues ready to be brought home.

3 large	egg whites	3 large
1 pinch	salt	1 pinch
½ t	white vinegar	3 mL
½ t	vanilla extract	3 mL
¼ C	sugar	60 mL
3 C	strawberries, hulled and sliced	750 mL
2 T	sugar	30 mL
2 C	low-fat frozen non-dairy whipped topping	500 mL

In a mixing bowl, beat the egg whites and salt until the whites hold stiff peaks. Beat in the vinegar, vanilla extract, and, very gradually, the sugar. Drop the mixture onto a well-greased cookie sheet, making nine equal circles about 3½ inches (10 cm) in diameter. Bake in a preheated 275° F (135° C) oven for 45 minutes. Remove to wire racks to cool. Meanwhile, in a mixing bowl, mix together the strawberries and sugar. Refrigerate until serving time. When ready to serve, place a meringue on each serving plate, put the strawberries on the meringue, and top with whipped topping.

Yield: 9 servings.
Each serving contains:

Calories (Kcal): 82

Carbohydrates (g): 16

Sodium (mg): 66

Diabetic exchange: 1 starch

Total fat (g): 0

Protein (g): 2

Cholesterol (mg): 0

Swiss Meringue Chantilly

Store these in airtight containers and they'll stay crisp for a day or two. Actually, my children like them mushy.

5 whole	egg whites	5 whole
¼ C	confectioners' sugar	60 mL
3½ T	cornstarch	50 mL
¼ C	confectioners' sugar	60 mL
2 C	low-fat frozen non-dairy whipped topping	500 mL
½ t	vanilla extract	3 mL
2 T	brandy (optional)	30 mL

Beat the egg whites in a large mixing bowl until they are stiff. Add the ¼ cup confectioners' sugar and the cornstarch and beat again. Fold in half the second batch of sugar. Line cookie sheets with flat pieces of brown paper (grocery) bags cut to fit, or use cooking parchment. Using a pastry bag, pipe 8 nests*. Bake in a preheated 250° F (120° C) oven for 1½ hours. The meringues will be dry. Peel the paper off the bottom. Just before serving, mix the frozen topping with the remaining sugar, vanilla extract, and the brandy, if desired. Spoon this mixture on top of the nests. Serve immediately.

* If you don't have a pastry bag, use a spoon to gently scoop the meringue into "nests."

Yield: 8 servings
Each serving contains:

Calories (Kcal): 85.3	Total fat (g): 0
Carbohydrates (g): 14.9	Protein (g): 2.2
Sodium (mg): 30	Cholesterol (mg): 0
Diabetic exchange: 1 starch	

Hungarian Cherry Pie

This is not a cherry pie in the gooey-filling tradition; it's more like pastry!

6 large	eggs, separated	6 large
¼ C	butter, margarine, or fat-free butter and oil replacement	60 mL
⅓ C	sugar	80 mL
½ whole	lemon peel, grated	½ whole
1 C	dry bread crumbs	250 mL
1 lb.	fresh sweet cherries, stemmed and pitted	450 g

In a mixing bowl cream together the egg yolks and butter. Gradually add half the sugar. In another bowl, beat the egg whites until foamy. Continue beating while adding the rest of the sugar. Beat the whites until stiff. Spoon a little of the egg whites on top of the yolk mixture. Gently fold the balance into the yolks. Sprinkle a third of the bread crumbs on top of the yolk mixture and fold together. Add more yolks and more bread crumbs and continue gently folding until they are all folded in. Pour the mixture into a well-greased pie pan. Scatter the cherries over the top of the mixture. Press them in lightly. Bake in a preheated 350° F (180° C) oven for 25 to 30 minutes. Serve hot, cut into wedges.

Yield: 12 servings.
Each serving contains:
Calories (Kcal): 146
Carbohydrates (g): 17
Sodium (mg): 133
Total fat (g): 7
Protein (g): 5
Cholesterol (mg): 116
Diabetic exchange: 1 starch; 1 fat

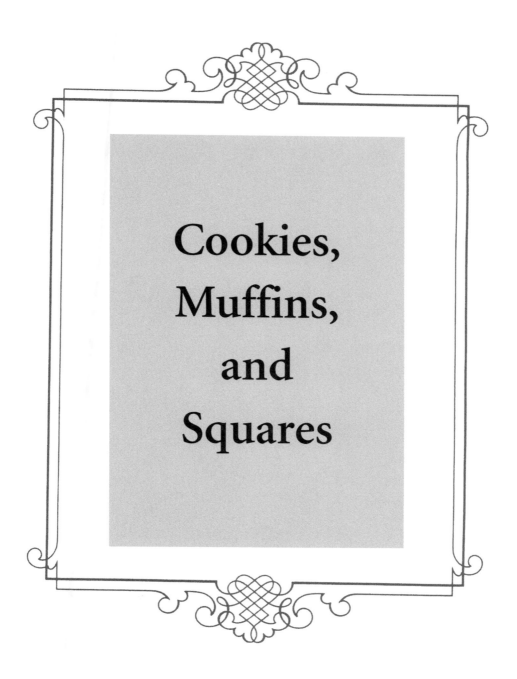

Cookies,
Muffins,
and
Squares

German Hazelnut Macaroons

Hazelnuts can be replaced by other nuts in this easy recipe.

2 large	egg whites	2 large
⅓ C	sugar	80 mL
1½ C	hazelnuts, shelled and ground	375 mL
6 T	unsweetened cocoa powder	90 mL
2 t	lemon peel, finely grated	10 mL
1 pinch	salt	1 pinch
1 t	vanilla extract	5 mL

In a large mixing bowl, beat the egg whites until they foam and thicken slightly. An electric mixer works best. Sprinkle the sugar over them and continue to beat until the whites form stiff peaks. In a small bowl, combine the ground hazelnuts, cocoa, lemon peel, salt, and vanilla extract. Fold the hazelnut mixture into the egg whites. Drop the dough by tablespoons onto well-greased baking sheets, spacing the macaroons about an inch (3 cm) apart. Set the sheets aside for an hour before baking.

Bake in the middle of a preheated 300° F (150° C) oven for 30 minutes. Cool on a rack and store in tightly sealed containers.

Yield: 44 cookies.
Each serving contains:

Calories (Kcal): 33
Carbohydrates (g): 3
Sodium (mg): 6
Diabetic exchange: ½ fat

Total fat (g): 3
Protein (g): 1
Cholesterol (mg): 0

Spanish Chocolate Meringue Cookies

One of my favorite taste-testers, Tim, loves these light and rich meringues. He says they're "fluffy and melt in your mouth."

4 large	egg whites	4 large
¼ t	cream of tartar	2 mL
1 pinch	salt	1 pinch
⅛ t	ground cinnamon	1 mL
½ t	vanilla extract	3 mL
⅓ C	sugar	80 mL
3 oz.	semisweet chocolate, finely grated	85 g

Beat the egg whites until they begin to foam. Add the cream of tartar and salt and continue to beat until the egg whites form stiff peaks. On medium speed, slowly add the cinnamon, vanilla extract, and sugar. Gradually add the chocolate. Spoon teaspoonfuls of meringue onto nonstick or well-greased cookie sheets. Bake in a 300° F (150° C) preheated oven. Bake for 25 to 30 minutes. The cookies will brown around the edges. Using a spatula, remove from cookie sheets and cool on a wire racks.

Yield: 70 cookies.
Each serving contains:

Calories (Kcal): 11	Total fat (g): 0
Carbohydrates (g): 0	Protein (g): 3
Sodium (mg): 9	Cholesterol (mg): 0
Diabetic exchange: free	

Chinese Almond Cookies

These are very like the almond cookies in Chinese restaurants. Very rich.

3 C	all-purpose flour, sifted	750 mL
4 T	almonds, finely chopped	60 mL
½ C	sugar	125 mL
½ t	salt	3 mL
2 t	baking soda	10 mL
1½ C	butter, margarine, or fat-free butter and oil replacement	375 mL
1 large	egg or equivalent egg substitute, lightly beaten	1 large
1 t	almond extract	5 mL
1 t	vanilla extract	5 mL

Mix the flour, almonds, sugar, salt, and baking soda together in a mixing bowl. Cut in the butter until the dough resembles coarse cornmeal. Add the egg, almond extract, and vanilla extract and blend. Form a ball from a piece of dough 1½ inches (5 cm) in diameter. Press the dough into a circle 1 inch (2.5 cm) in diameter. Continue until all the dough has been used. Place the cookies on well-greased cookie sheets ½ inch (3 cm) apart and bake in a preheated 350° F (180° C) oven for 12 minutes.

Yield: 72 cookies.
Each serving contains:

Calories (Kcal): 62	Total fat (g): 4
Carbohydrates (g): 6	Protein (g): 1
Sodium (mg): 89	Cholesterol (mg): 13
Diabetic exchange: 1 fat	

German Dark Pfefferneusse Cookies

If you want more of a bite, add more pepper. Freshly ground pepper really is the best.

3 T	brown sugar, packed	45 mL
3 T	dark corn syrup	45 mL
4 T	lowfat 1% milk	60 mL
2 T	butter, margarine, or fat-free butter and oil replacement	30 mL
1 large	egg or equivalent egg substitute, lightly beaten	1 large
½ t	anise extract	3 mL
¼ t	baking powder	2 mL
⅛ t	vanilla extract	1 mL
⅛ t	ground cloves	1 mL
⅛ t	ground cardamom	1 mL
⅛ t	salt	1 mL
1 dash	pepper	1 dash
2½ C	flour	625 mL
3 T	powdered sugar	45 mL

In a saucepan, mix the brown sugar, corn syrup, milk, and shortening and heat to boiling. Cool. Beat in the egg. Add the anise extract, baking powder, vanilla extract, cloves, cardamom, salt, and pepper. Mix well. Mix in enough of the flour, a cup at a time, to make a very stiff dough, kneading in the last addition. Dust a work surface with the powdered sugar. Shape the dough into rolls ¾ inch (3 cm) thick. Cut each roll in pieces ¾ inch (3 cm) long. Arrange on an ungreased cookie sheet in a preheated 375° F (190° C) oven until brown, 8–12 minutes. Cool 1 to 2 minutes before removing from the cookie sheet.

Yield: 96 cookies.
Each serving contains:

Calories (Kcal): 19
Carbohydrates (g): 4
Sodium (mg): 8
Diabetic exchange: free

Total fat (g): 0
Protein (g): 0
Cholesterol (mg): 3

Italian Fig Cookies

The little "figlets" are fine in this recipe too; just be sure they aren't sweetened.

1½ C	figs, dried	225 g
¾ C	raisins	115 g
¼ C	slivered almonds	35 g
2 T	sugar	30 mL
¼ C	hot water	60 mL
¼ t	ground cinnamon	2 mL
1 dash	pepper	1 dash
2½ C	all-purpose flour	625 mL
¼ C	sugar	60 mL
¼ t	baking powder	2 mL
10 T	butter, margarine, or fat-free butter and oil replacement	150 mL
½ C	lowfat 1% milk	125 mL
1 large	egg or equivalent egg substitute, beaten	1 large

Chop figs, raisins, and almonds together in a food processor. In a mixing bowl combine the 2 T (30 mL) sugar, hot water, cinnamon, and pepper. Add the chopped-fruit mixture. Set aside. In another mixing bowl, combine the flour, ¼ cup sugar, and baking powder. Cut in the butter and blend until the pieces are the size of small peas. Stir in the milk and egg until all the dry mixture is moistened. Divide the dough in half. On a lightly floured work surface roll each half into an 18 × 16-inch (46 × 40 cm) rectangle. Cut each rectangle into four strips 18 × 4 inches (46 × 10 cm). Spread about ⅓ cup (80 mL) of the fig mixture over each strip of dough. Roll the dough up jelly-roll fashion, starting at the long side. Cut each filled strip into six 3-inch (8 cm) lengths. Place the cookies, seam-side down, on ungreased cookie sheets. Curve each cookie slightly. Snip the outer edge of the curve three times. Bake in a preheated 350° F (180° C) oven until lightly browned, 20 to 25 minutes. Remove from cookie sheets and cool on a rack.

Yield: 24 large cookies.
Each serving contains:
Calories (Kcal): 161   Total fat (g): 6
Carbohydrates (g): 25   Protein (g): 3
Sodium (mg): 60   Cholesterol (mg): 22
Diabetic exchange: 1 starch; 1 fruit; ½ fat

Chinese Sweet Crescents

Make sure your oil is really hot before you start cooking or else these crescents will be greasy and soggy.

½ C	salted peanuts, chopped	75g
½ C	coconut flakes	35 g
¼ C	brown sugar	60 mL
¼ C	granulated sugar	60 mL
1 pkg.	wonton wrappers	1 pkg.
1 large	egg, or equivalent egg substitute, beaten	1 large

Mix peanuts, coconut, brown sugar, and granulated sugar. Fold a wonton square in half, then in half again into a square. Fold once more to make a triangle. Round off the top corner, the one away from the center, with scissors. This makes a circle. Place 1 teaspoon of the filling in the center. Moisten edges with beaten egg, fold in half, and seal to make a half circle. Deep fry in hot oil until golden, turning once. Drain. Cool. Store in an airtight container.

Yield: 72 cookies.
Each serving contains:
Calories (Kcal): 14
Carbohydrates (g): 2
Sodium (mg): 3
Diabetic exchange: free

Total fat (g): 0
Protein (g): 0
Cholesterol (mg): 3

Middle Eastern Date Pastry

These are actually little cookies that melt in your mouth. They keep well in a tightly closed container.

Pastry

1¾ C	flour	435 mL
7 T	butter, margarine, or fat-free butter and oil replacement	350 mL
1 T	confectioner's sugar	15 mL
1 T	canola oil	15 mL
2 T	lowfat 1% milk	30 mL

Filling

1 ⅓ C	dates, pitted	330 mL
1 T	butter, margarine, or fat-free butter and oil replacement	15 mL
3 T	water	45 mL

Cut the butter into the flour, using a pair of knives, a pastry blender, or a food processor. Add the sugar. Mix well. Make a well and pour in the oil and milk. Knead for 10 minutes. Wrap in plastic wrap and place in the refrigerator while you make the filling.

Chop the dates fine, using a food processor. Heat the dates, butter, and water in a heavy-base frying pan over low heat, stirring and pressing until a paste forms. Cool.

Grease and flour a baking sheet, shaking off the excess flour. Cut the dough into three pieces. Knead each piece and roll out as thinly as possible into a rectangle. Spread one-third of the filling onto each rectangle, leaving a ⅜-inch (1 cm) border of uncovered pastry all around. Roll it up from one end. Continue rolling backward and forward, pressing down lightly to lengthen the roll. Slightly flatten each roll using your hands. Slice diagonally into pieces about ¾ inch (2 cm) thick. Place the slices on a baking sheet. Prick the tops lightly with a fork.

Bake in a preheated 350° F (180° C) oven for 20 to 30 minutes. The pastry should be white on top and slightly browned underneath. Sprinkle with confectioner's sugar, if desired. Remove to a cooling rack.

Yield: 36 pastries.
Each serving contains:

Calories (Kcal): 65	Total fat (g): 3
Carbohydrates (g): 10	Protein (g): 1
Sodium (mg): 230	Cholesterol (mg): 6

Diabetic exchange: ½ fruit; ½ fat

British Strawberry Muffins

Don't skip toasting the muffin halves before you serve these strawberry muffins. The crunchiness makes a real difference.

Muffins

½ cup	flour	250 mL
pinch	salt	pinch
2 t	sugar	10 mL
1¼ C	lowfat 1% milk, warmed	310 mL
2 t	dry yeast	10 mL
1 large	egg or equivalent egg substitute, well beaten	1 large
1 T	butter, margarine, or fat-free replacement, melted	15 mL

Topping

1 lb.	strawberries, sliced	450 g
1 C	low-fat frozen non-dairy whipped topping	250 mL

Combine the flour and salt in a mixing bowl. In another small bowl, combine the sugar, milk, and yeast. Stir well and put in a warm, draft-free place for 10 minutes. Add the yeast mixture to the flour mixture along with the egg. Stir in the melted butter, and knead for 10 minutes. It will make a soft dough. Turn the dough into an oiled bowl, cover with plastic wrap or a tea towel and put in a warm, draft-free place to rise until doubled in bulk (approximately an hour or so). Turn out the dough onto a lightly floured work surface, punch down the dough, and, using a rolling pin, roll out until it is ½ inch (1.5 cm) thick. Cut 3-inch (7.5 cm) rounds. Put each round onto a floured work surface, dust with flour, and cover with plastic wrap or a tea towel until doubled in bulk. Heat a heavy-bottomed frying pan or griddle. Grease lightly and fry the muffins to cook them, about eight minutes on each side. Before serving, mix the sliced strawberries and whipped topping. When ready to serve, split the muffins in half, toast both sides, and place strawberries on top of each half.

Yield: 12 servings.
Each serving contains:

Calories (Kcal): 181	Total fat (g): 2
Carbohydrates (g): 33	Protein (g): 6
Sodium (mg): 47	Cholesterol (mg): 21

Diabetic exchange: 2 starch; 1 fruit

Middle Eastern Farina and Date Bars

The farina in this recipe tastes like toasted sesame seeds.

8 oz.	dates, pitted	225 g
¼ C	butter or fat-free butter and oil replacement	60 mL
⅔ C	farina	165 mL

Chop the dates into tiny pieces (a food processor works well). Mix with the butter and work into a paste using a damp knife or a food processor. Dry-roast the farina in a heavy frying pan, stirring constantly. As soon as it begins to color and smell roasted, remove from the heat so it doesn't burn. Continue to stir. Return to very low heat to try for even color. Be very careful not to burn the farina. Mix the farina with the date paste. Roll thinly between 2 sheets of waxed paper. Use a sharp knife with a wet blade to cut into diamond shapes 1 inch (3 cm) wide. Separate them, peel off from the waxed paper, and leave to dry out in a cool place.

Yield: 48 servings.
Each serving contains:

Calories (Kcal): 30

Carbohydrates (g): 5

Sodium (mg): 10

Diabetic exchange: free

Total fat (g): 1

Protein (g): 0

Cholesterol (mg): 3

Polish Apple Squares

These squares hold together very nicely and are a great alternative to brownies.

1¾ C	all-purpose flour	435 mL
¼ C	sugar	60 mL
2 t	baking powder	10 mL
¼ C	butter, margarine, or fat-free butter and oil replacement	60 mL
½ C	fat-free cream cheese	125 mL
2 large	eggs or equivalent egg substitute, lightly beaten	2 large
1 C	fat-free sour cream	250 mL
1 t	vanilla extract	5 mL
1½ lbs.	cooking apples	680 g
½ C	raisins	125 mL
2 T	sugar	30 mL
1 t	cinnamon	5 mL
1 t	vanilla extract	5 mL

Stir together the flour, sugar, and baking powder. In a mixing bowl, cut in the butter until the pieces resemble small peas. In another bowl, combine the eggs, sour cream, and vanilla extract. Pour this over the flour mixture and stir until well mixed. Spread half the batter into a well-greased 9 × 9 × 2-inch (23 × 23 × 4 cm) baking pan. Bake in a preheated 350° F (180° C) oven for 15 minutes. Peel, core, and finely chop the apples. In a large mixing bowl, combine the apples, raisins, sugar, cinnamon, and vanilla extract. Spread the apple mixture over the cooked batter. Carefully top with the remaining batter. Bake in a 350° F (180° C) preheated oven for 35 minutes. Cut into squares.

Yield: 16 servings.
Each serving contains:

Calories (Kcal): 158

Carbohydrates (g): 27

Sodium (mg): 117

Total fat (g): 4

Protein (g): 3

Cholesterol (mg): 36

Diabetic exchange: 1 starch; 1 fruit; ½ fat

Brazilian Peanut Squares

One of my friend Cristina Junqueira's favorite recipes from her home in Brazil.

8 large	eggs, separated	8 large
½ C	sugar	125 mL
6 T	flour	90 mL
1 C	unsalted roasted peanuts, chopped	250 mL
1 T	sugar	15 mL
1 t	cinnamon	5 mL

In a large mixing bowl, beat the egg whites until foamy. Continue beating until stiff. In another bowl, gradually beat the yolks together with the sugar until the batter is smooth and creamy. Add the flour and beat again. Mix the chopped peanuts into the batter. Fold in the egg whites. Pour into a well-greased and floured 8½ x 8½-inch (28 × 21 cm) square pan. Bake in a preheated 375° F (190° C) oven for 25 minutes or until a toothpick inserted into the center comes out clean. Cool on a wire rack. Cut into 16 squares. In a teacup mix together the 1 T (15 mL) of sugar and the cinnamon. Put the sugar and cinnamon mixture on a piece of waxed paper. While warm, roll each of the squares in it.

Yield: 16 servings.
Each serving contains:
Calories (Kcal): 128
Carbohydrates (g): 11
Sodium (mg): 32
Total fat (g): 7
Protein (g): 6
Cholesterol (mg): 106
Diabetic exchange: 1 starch; 1 fat

German Gingerbread

Chocolate underscores the traditional gingerbread spices in this moist ginger-bread.

2 oz.	unsweetened chocolate squares	60 g
4 T	butter, margarine, or fat-free replacement, at room temperature	60 mL
⅓ C	sugar	80 mL
3 large	eggs, whites only	3 large
1 C	fat-free cream cheese	250 mL
2 C	all-purpose flour	500 mL
1 T	ground cinnamon	15 mL
1 T	ground allspice	15 mL
1 T	ground cloves	15 mL
¼ t	ground nutmeg	2 mL
1 t	baking powder	5 mL
¼ t	salt	2 mL
1 t	vanilla extract	5 mL
1 C	pecans, chopped fine (optional)	250 mL

In a heavy-bottomed saucepan or the top of a double boiler, melt the chocolate. Set aside to cool. In a large mixing bowl beat the butter, adding the sugar gradually. Beat until creamy. Add the egg whites, one at a time, and beat well after each. Beat in the cream cheese and the cooled chocolate. Add the flour, spices, and salt, then add the vanilla extract and nuts, if desired. Beat until combined. Pour the batter into a well-greased 9-inch (23 cm) square baking pan. Bake in a preheated 350° F (180° C) oven for 40 minutes. The top will spring back when pressed lightly. Place pan on wire rack to cool.

Yield: 9 servings.
Each serving contains:

Calories (Kcal): 182	Total fat (g): 7
Carbohydrates (g): 26	Protein (g): 5
Sodium (mg): 186	Cholesterol (mg): 14

Diabetic exchange: 1 whole milk; 1 fruit

Greek Rusks

Like most rusk recipes from around the world, these are baked twice, the last time to make them crisp.

¼ C	butter	60 mL
1 t	vanilla extract	5 mL
⅓ C	sugar	80 mL
3 large	eggs, or equivalent egg substitute	3 large
1 large	egg yolk	1 large
3½ C	cake flour, sifted	875 mL
1 T	baking powder	45 mL
¼ t	salt	2 mL
1 large	egg yolk, lightly beaten	1 large

In a mixing bowl beat the butter, vanilla extract, and sugar until fluffy. Add the eggs, one at a time, beating for a minute after each addition. In another bowl, combine the flour, baking powder, and salt. Mix well. Pour half the flour mixture into the butter mixture. Mix well. Add the remaining flour. Mix well.

Divide the dough into four portions. On a well-floured work surface, roll each part into a long roll about 1½ inches in diameter. Place the rolls on a well-greased and floured cookie sheet. Flatten the dough slightly. Brush the tops with the egg yolk.

Bake in a preheated 400° F (200° C) oven for about 20 minutes. The dough will be golden and firm to the touch. Cover with a tea towel and cool on racks for at least two hours. Cut the rolls into ½-inch (3 cm) slices. Place on an ungreased cookie sheet, cut-side down. Bake in a preheated 400° F (200° C) oven for 15 to 20 minutes, turning several times.

Yield: 36 rusks.
Each serving contains:

Calories (Kcal): 66	Total fat (g): 1
Carbohydrates (g): 10	Protein (g): 1
Sodium (mg): 64	Cholesterol (mg): 33
Diabetic exchange: 1 starch	

Japanese Bean Paste Cakes

For a more traditional flavor use azuki beans.

1 C	canned kidney beans, drained	250 mL
¼ C	sugar	60 mL
2¼ C	flour	560 mL
3 t	baking powder	15 mL
½ t	salt	3 mL
¼ C	sugar	60 mL
1½ T	butter, margarine, or fat-free butter and oil replacement	17 mL
¼ C	water	60 mL

Blend the beans and sugar in a blender or food processor, adding a little water if needed to make a thick paste. Sift the flour, baking powder, salt, and additional sugar together. Cut in the butter until the mixture is well blended. Add the water a little at a time until the dough is soft but not sticky. Place the dough on a well-floured work surface and knead a few minutes. Shape the dough into 1½-inch (5 cm) balls. Flatten each piece of dough and spoon ¾ teaspoon of bean paste into the center. Fold the dough around the filling. Place the filled cakes upside down on a piece of waxed paper. Steam, covered, for 15 minutes. Serve cold.

Yield: 22 cakes.
Each serving contains:
Calories (Kcal): 99
Carbohydrates (g): 19
Sodium (mg): 108
Diabetic exchange: 1 starch

Total fat (g): 1
Protein (g): 3
Cholesterol (mg): 2

Fruit

Swedish Baked Apples with Almond Topping

In Sweden, this popular dessert is actually called "French applesauce."

2 C	cold water	500 mL
¼ whole	lemon (separate and chop the peel; reserve the piece of lemon)	¼ whole
4 large	tart green cooking apples, halved, peeled, and cored	4 large
4 T	butter, margarine, or fat-free replacement	60 mL
¼ C	sugar	60 mL
3 large	egg yolks or equivalent egg substitute	3 large
½ t	almond extract	3 mL
½ C	almonds, blanched and ground	125 mL
2 t	lemon juice	10 mL
3 large	egg whites	3 large
1 pinch	salt	1 pinch
dollop	frozen non-dairy whipped topping (optional)	dollop

Put the water into a two-quart (2 L) saucepan. Squeeze the lemon piece and put the juice into the water and toss in the pieces of lemon peel. Add the apple halves. Bring the water to a boil, lower the heat, and simmer for five minutes or longer, until the apples are tender. Carefully remove the apples halves from the pan and drain them on a cake rack. Place them in a single layer, cut-side down, side by side in a greased shallow baking dish. Preheat the oven to 350° F (180° C). In a mixing bowl, cream the butter until smooth. Beat in the sugar slowly, then add the egg yolks one at a time. Add the almond extract, then add the almonds and lemon juice. In a larger mixing bowl, beat the egg whites with the pinch of salt until stiff peaks form. Fold 2 tablespoons (30 mL) of stiff egg whites into the butter mixture. With a rubber spatula, gently fold the butter mixture into the stiffly beaten egg whites. Spread the topping lightly over the apples and bake for about 20 minutes, until the surface turns golden. Serve at room temperature, with whipped topping if desired.

Yield: 8 servings.
Each serving contains:

Calories (Kcal): 188	Total fat (g): 12
Carbohydrates (g): 17	Protein (g): 4
Sodium (mg): 102	Cholesterol (mg): 95

Diabetic exchange: 1 starch; 2 fat

Irish Stuffed Baked Apples

These apples served warm are a lovely winter dessert. Serve cool in the hotter months.

4 whole	cooking apples (i.e., Rome Beauties)	4 whole
½ C	whole-berry cranberry sauce	125 mL
1 C	unsweetened apple juice	250 mL
1 T	low-fat frozen non-dairy whipped topping	15 mL

Wash and core the apples. Peel the skin on the top half of each apple to prevent splitting. Place apples upright in small baking dish. Fill cavities in apples with cranberry sauce. Pour apple cider around apples and cover the whole pan tightly with aluminum foil. Bake in a preheated 375° F (190° C) oven for 30–40 minutes. Serve with whipped topping.

Yield: 4 servings.
Each serving contains:

Calories (Kcal): 136

Carbohydrates (g): 35

Sodium (mg): 11

Diabetic exchange: 2 fruit

Total fat (g): 0

Protein (g): 0

Cholesterol (mg): 0

Latvian Poached Apples

I had these for a luncheon dessert in Latvia—in a fairytale castle in the countryside outside Riga. Our fabulous hostess, Inez, from the Latvian Friendship Society, made sure that every meal was a window to her culture.

2 C	unsweetened apple juice	500 mL
16 whole	cloves	16 whole
4 large	green cooking apples, peeled and cored	4 large
8 T	light chocolate syrup	120 mL
1 C	low-fat frozen non-dairy whipped topping	250 mL

In a large, heavy saucepan, bring the apple juice to a boil. Insert four cloves around the top of each of the apples. Put the apples side by side in the saucepan. Spoon some apple juice over the apples to baste them. Turn the heat to low, cover the pan, and simmer for 15 minutes or so. You'll need to baste a few times during the 15 minutes. If the apples are not tender, cook for a few more minutes until they are. Leave them in the juice to cool. Discard the cooking juice. To serve, swirl 1 tablespoon (15 mL) of syrup on each of the four serving plates. Arrange an apple on each plate and top with whipped topping. Drizzle the remaining chocolate syrup over the top.

Yield: 4 servings.
Each serving contains:
Calories (Kcal): 144
Carbohydrates (g): 32
Sodium (mg): 23
Diabetic exchange: 2 fruit

Total fat (g): 0
Protein (g): 0
Cholesterol (mg): 0

Polish Apple Charlotte

I use the frozen prepared pie crusts—they are so handy.

10 large	apples	10 large
	sugar, to taste (optional)	
	cinnamon, to taste (optional)	
1 T	butter, margarine, or fat-free replacement	15 mL
2 T	all-fruit apricot jam	30 mL
2 T	seedless raisins	30 mL
1 whole	frozen pie crust	1 whole

Core and pare the apples and slice them thin. Combine apples, sugar, cinnamon, and butter in a heavy-bottomed saucepan. Cover tightly and simmer for about 10 minutes. Add the jam and raisins and mix thoroughly. Pour the apple mixture into the prepared pie crust and bake in a 400° F (200° C) oven for 30 to 40 minutes.

Yield: 12 servings.
Each serving contains:
Calories (Kcal): 143   Total fat (g): 5
Carbohydrates (g): 26   Protein (g): 1
Sodium (mg): 78   Cholesterol (mg): 3
Diabetic exchange: 2 fruit; 1 fat

Polish Rice and Apples in Froth

The "froth" is a meringue top for a moist apple filling. I use dried packaged egg whites.

1 C	rice	250 mL
2 C	lowfat 1% milk	500 mL
4 whole	eggs, separated	4 whole
3 T	sugar	45 mL
1 t	bread crumbs	5 mL
4 T	all-fruit raspberry jam	60 mL
2 large	apples, peeled and sliced	2 large
6 large	egg whites	6 large
2 T	sugar	30 mL

Put the rice and milk in a heavy-bottomed saucepan and cook until the rice is tender. Set aside to cool. Put the egg yolks in a mixing bowl and beat with sugar until light and creamy. Combine the yolk mixture and rice in the bowl. Beat the four whites until stiff and fold into the rice mixture. Grease an 8- or 9-inch (21–23 cm) cake pan and coat with bread crumbs.

Bake in a 350° F (165 ° C) oven for 30 minutes. Remove to rack. Cool. Turn out of pan and spread with the jam. Cover with the apples. Beat the six egg whites and sugar until stiff, and cover the apples with this mixture. Bake in 400° F (200° C) for 15–20 minutes. The top should be light brown.

Yield: 8 servings.
Each serving contains:

Calories (Kcal): 236	Total fat (g): 4
Carbohydrates (g): 41	Protein (g): 10
Sodium (mg): 107	Cholesterol (mg): 109

Diabetic exchange: 1 lowfat milk; 2 fruit

Portuguese Pineapple in Port with Fresh Chopped Mint

Pineapples came to Portugal in the 15th century. This is a delightful and easy recipe.

20 oz.	pineapple chunks in juice	570 grams
3 T	Port wine	45 mL
¼ C	fresh mint, minced	60 mL

Drain the juice from the pineapple and place the wedges in a large non-metallic bowl. Add the Port and toss to mix. Cover with plastic wrap and chill for three to four hours. Add the mint, toss again, and chill for 30 minutes longer. Serve in glass dessert dishes.

Yield: 6 servings.
Each serving contains:

Calories (Kcal): 68
Carbohydrates (g): 15
Sodium (mg): 1
Diabetic exchange: 1 fruit

Total fat (g): 0
Protein (g): 0
Cholesterol (mg): 0

Jamaican Pineapple Fool

You can use canned pineapple, but it's not as good.

2 C	fresh pineapple, finely chopped	500 mL
2 C	low-fat frozen non-dairy whipped topping	500 mL

Just before serving, mix the ingredients together and spoon into individual serving dishes.

Yield: 4 servings.
Each serving contains:
Calories (Kcal): 102
Carbohydrates (g): 17.6
Sodium (mg): 41
Diabetic exchange: 1 fruit

Total fat (g): 0.3
Protein (g): 0.3
Cholesterol (mg): 0

Martinique Baked Bananas with Cream Cheese

Nothing can describe how wonderful this smells bubbling in your oven.

8 oz.	fat-free cream cheese, softened	225 grams
3 T	light brown sugar, sifted	45 mL
¾ t	ground cinnamon	4 mL
2 T	butter, margarine, or fat-free replacement	60 mL
6 large	bananas, firm, cut in half lengthwise	6 large
¼ C	low-fat frozen non-dairy whipped topping	60 mL

In a large mixing bowl, cream together the cheese, sugar, and ½ teaspoon of the cinnamon until light and fluffy. In a skillet or frying pan, melt half the butter over moderate heat. Add one or two banana halves, and brown lightly on both sides. Turn them gently with a spatula, regulating the heat so that they color evenly without burning. Transfer the cooked bananas to a plate and set them aside while you brown the remaining ones in the remaining butter. Arrange the banana halves in a single layer, cut-side down, in a shallow baking dish large enough to hold them easily. Spread half the cream cheese mixture on top. Arrange a layer of the bananas on top. Spread them with the rest of the cream cheese. Pour the whipped topping over the top and bake in a preheated 350° F (180° C) oven for half an hour or so until the bananas are tender but still intact and the sauce is golden brown. Sprinkle with the remaining ¼ teaspoon (2 mL) of cinnamon. Serve warm.

Yield: 6 servings.
Each serving contains:

Calories (Kcal): 146	Total fat (g): 3
Carbohydrates (g): 26	Protein (g): 3
Sodium (mg): 118	Cholesterol (mg): 13

Diabetic exchange: 1 starch; 1 fruit; ½ fat

Central American Plantains with Cream

I always look for these on menus in Cuban restaurants. Use bananas if you can't get plantains.

3 T	butter or margarine	45 mL
2 T	brown sugar	30 mL
1 t	vanilla	5 mL
¼ t	cinnamon	2 mL
2 C	sliced bananas or plantains	500 mL
¼ C	low-fat frozen non-dairy whipped topping	60 mL
2 T	toasted slivered almonds	30 mL

Melt the butter over low heat in a large skillet. Add the brown sugar, vanilla, and cinnamon. Stir. Add the bananas and stir gently to coat. Remove from heat. Spoon into four serving bowls. Top with whipped topping and almonds.

Yield: 4 servings.
Each serving contains:
Calories (Kcal): 231.2   Total fat (g): 11.3
Carbohydrates (g): 32.9   Protein (g): 2.2
Sodium (mg): 95   Cholesterol (mg): 23
Diabetic exchange: 2 starch; 1 fat

Mexican Baked Plantains with Prunes

This recipe only works with plantains. Bananas won't substitute. Look for plantains in the exotic fruit section of the grocery store.

3 large	ripe plantains	3 large
1 C	prunes, pitted and chopped	250 mL
½ C	fresh orange juice	125 mL
1 T	fresh lime juice	15 mL
3 T	dark rum	45 mL
2 T	sugar	30 mL
2 T	butter	30 mL
½ C	non-fat yogurt	125 mL
2 T	low-fat 1% milk	30 mL
3 t	honey	15 mL

Place the unpeeled plantains in a well-greased baking dish. Bake in a pre-heated 350° F (180° C) for 30 minutes, until the skin is blackened and split. Remove the plantains from the oven and let cool. When cooled, peel the plantains and cut off the ends. Slice lengthwise and remove the tough inner core. Cut into 2-inch (5 cm) pieces. Return the pieces to the baking dish and toss with the prunes.

In a small bowl, combine the orange juice, lime juice, rum, and sugar. Stir this mixture until the sugar is dissolved, and spoon over the plantains. Dot with the butter and cover the baking dish tightly with foil. Bake in a preheated 350° F (180° C) oven for 20 minutes. The plantains should be fork-tender. To make the topping, beat together the yogurt, milk, and honey in a small bowl. Serve the plantains and prunes warm, topped with the flavored yogurt.

Yield: 8 servings.
Each serving contains:

Calories (Kcal): 204	Total fat (g): 3.3
Carbohydrates (g): 56.6	Protein (g): 2.5
Sodium (mg): 61	Cholesterol (mg): 8.2

Diabetic exchange: 1 starch; 2 fruit

Italian Fresh Fruit Dessert

What could be more delightful on a summer evening? Make this ahead of time and chill it.

1 C	seedless grapes	250 mL
1 C	pineapple chunks in water, drained	250 mL
1 C	cantaloupe, cut into cubes	250 mL
1 C	honeydew melon, cut into cubes	250 mL
¼ C	fresh mint leaves, chopped	60 mL
½ C	marsala wine	125 mL

Cut fruit into small pieces. Combine ingredients in a serving bowl. Toss lightly.

Yield: 6 servings.
Each serving contains:

Calories (Kcal): 66
Carbohydrates (g): 13
Sodium (mg): 11
Diabetic exchange: 1 fruit

Total fat (g): 0
Protein (g): 1
Cholesterol (mg): 0

Mexican Fruit Ambrosia

A delicious summertime treat—better than ice cream.

2 C	fresh pineapple, chopped	500 mL
1 whole	papaya, peeled, seeded, and chopped	1 whole
2 C	strawberries, hulled and quartered	500 mL
2 whole	nectarines, peeled, pitted, and chopped	2 whole
¼ C	flaked coconut	60 mL
2 T	honey	30 mL
¼ C	tequila	60 mL
¼ C	fresh lime juice	60 mL

In a large serving bowl, combine the pineapple, papaya, strawberries, nectarines, and coconut flakes. In a small bowl, stir together the honey, tequila, and lime juice. Toss the honey mixture with the fruit. Cover and refrigerate for 1 hour before serving.

Yield: 6 servings.
Each serving contains:
Calories (Kcal): 142.5
Carbohydrates (g): 28.4
Sodium (mg): 11
Diabetic exchange: 1 starch; 1 fruit

Total fat (g): 1.7
Protein (g): 1.4
Cholesterol (mg): 0

German Beer Fruit Cup

You'll be pleasantly surprised how nicely refreshing this fruit cup is on a summer day.

1 C	strawberries, hulled and quartered	250 mL
2 slices	canned pineapple	2 slices
2 whole	oranges, peeled and cut into segments	2 whole
4 C	beer	1 L

Put the fruit into a deep mixing bowl. Stir to combine. Add the beer to cover. Marinate, stirring occasionally, for 12 hours.

Yield: 6 servings.
Each serving contains:

Calories (Kcal): 107	Total fat (g): 0.2
Carbohydrates (g): 16.4	Protein (g): 1.3
Sodium (mg): 8	Cholesterol (mg): 0
Diabetic exchange: 1 starch	

South Pacific Baked Tropical Fruits

Fresh pineapple is the best, but canned is okay, too.

3 C	pineapple chunks in water, diced	750 mL
2 C	mango, diced	500 mL
2 C	papaya, diced	500 mL
3 medium	bananas, sliced	3 medium
½ C	cornstarch	125 mL
1 t	vanilla extract	5 mL
2 T	brown sugar	30 mL
1½ C	low-fat frozen non-dairy whipped topping	375 mL
1 t	coconut extract	5 mL

Put the fruit in a food processor or blender. Purée, pouring the juice into a saucepan as it accumulates. When you have at least one cup of juice in the saucepan, add the cornstarch and blend it into the juice using a whisk. Add the rest of the fruit purée and cook over medium heat, stirring constantly until the mixture thickens. Add the vanilla extract and brown sugar. Stir well and continue to cook until the sugar is dissolved. Pour into a well-greased serving dish. Chill. The fruit will congeal further as it cools. Before serving, blend the coconut extract thoroughly into whipped topping. Garnish each serving with a dollop of the coconut-flavored whipped topping.

Yield: 12 servings.
Each serving contains:

Calories (Kcal): 116	Total fat (g): 0
Carbohydrates (g): 27	Protein (g): 1
Sodium (mg): 13	Cholesterol (mg): 0
Diabetic exchange: 2 fruit	

Mexican Blueberries and Papaya

Traditional Mexican papaya, with the contemporary touch of blueberries, makes a dessert that's as beautiful as it is delicious.

2 medium	papayas, quartered, seeded, and peeled	2 medium
1 T	sugar	15 mL
¼ C	fresh lime juice	60 mL
¾ C	blueberries	185 mL

Put the papayas into a food processor or blender. Add the sugar and lime juice and purée until smooth. Pour into a shallow serving bowl. Refrigerate. Just before serving, stir the papaya mixture, then carefully spoon the blueberries onto the top.

Yield: 6 servings.
Each serving contains:

Calories (Kcal): 60.5
Carbohydrates (g): 15.5
Sodium (mg): 4
Diabetic exchange: 1 fruit

Total fat (g): 0.2
Protein (g): 0.8
Cholesterol (mg): 0

Dominican Republic Papaya Frappé

A lovely, cooling drink.

1 medium	papaya, peeled, seeded, and chopped	1 medium
½ C	low-fat 1% milk	125 mL
3 T	fresh lime juice	45 mL
½ t	lime zest	3 mL
2 T	sugar	30 mL
½ t	vanilla extract	3 mL
½ C	crushed ice cubes	125 mL

Put the papaya into a blender or food processor, add the rest of the ingredients, and blend at a high speed for 30 seconds. The papaya should be completely puréed. Serve at once in tall glasses.

Yield: 2 servings.
Each serving contains:
Calories (Kcal): 140.6
Carbohydrates (g): 32.6
Sodium (mg): 37
Diabetic exchange: 2 fruit

Total fat: 0.9
Protein (g): 3.1
Cholesterol (mg): 37

German Peach-Apricot Dessert

I love this dish. It can be thrown together on the spur of the moment, and by the time you take it out of the oven you can have dinner ready, too!

32 oz.	peaches, packed in juice	900 g
8 oz.	dried apricot halves	230 g
1	juice of orange	1
½	orange peel, do not chop	½
½ C	gingersnap cookies, crumbled	125 mL
¼ C	brown sugar, packed	60 mL
1 C	fat-free sour cream	250 mL

Drain the peaches, saving one cup of the juice. In a medium baking dish, combine peaches, cup of reserved juice, apricots, orange juice, and orange peel. Gently arrange the crumbled gingersnaps on top of the fruit, gently pressing into the fruit. Sprinkle brown sugar over the gingersnaps. Bake in a preheated 350° F (180° C) oven, uncovered, for one hour, or until the fruit mixture is thickened and somewhat caramelized. Serve hot, topped with sour cream.

Yield: 8 servings.
Each serving contains:
Calories (Kcal): 214   Total fat (g): 2
Carbohydrates (g): 51   Protein (g): 4
Sodium (mg): 126   Cholesterol (mg): 2
Diabetic exchange: 1 starch; 2 fruit

Polish Kompot A Suszu

A "fruit soup" you make from a bag of dried fruit; I serve it cold in the summer.

8 oz.	dried mixed fruit	225 g
2½ C	water	625 mL
2 T	sugar	30 mL
1 t	lemon peel, grated	5 mL
1 T	lemon juice	15 mL
2 sticks	cinnamon	2 sticks
6 T	low-fat frozen non-dairy whipped topping	90 mL

With a pair of scissors, cut up the large pieces of fruit. Put them into a saucepan with the water. Bring to a boil over medium heat. Reduce heat, cover, and simmer for 30 to 35 minutes. Add the rest of the ingredients. Stir. Simmer for 10 more minutes. Chill. Garnish with a dollop of whipped topping when serving.

Yield: 6 servings.
Each serving contains:

Calories (Kcal): 68

Carbohydrates (g): 16

Sodium (mg): 16

Diabetic exchange: 1 fruit

Total fat (g): 0

Protein (g): 1

Cholesterol (mg): 0

Iranian Fresh Melon and Peach Compote

Frozen melon balls are fine in this recipe, but don't use canned peaches.

1 medium	Persian melon	1 medium
½ t	salt	3 mL
3 medium	peaches, peeled and sliced	3 medium
¼ C	sugar	60 mL
3 T	lemon juice	45 mL
2 T	rosewater	30 mL

Make melon balls from the fleshy part of the melon. Save any juice. Put the melon balls and the juice in a bowl and toss with the salt. Add the rest of the ingredients and toss to combine. Cover and refrigerate until thoroughly chilled before serving.

Yield: 6 servings.
Each serving contains:
Calories (Kcal): 128
Carbohydrates (g): 34
Sodium (mg): 199
Diabetic exchange: 2 fruit

Total fat (g): 0
Protein (g): 1
Cholesterol (mg): 0

French Flamed Peaches

This is so very impressive a flaming desert, it's the perfect end to a meal.

4 whole	peaches, ripe, peeled and cut into slices	4 whole
2 T	lemon juice	30 mL
1 T	unsalted butter	15 mL
2 T	sugar	30 mL
2 T	brandy	30 mL

Sprinkle the peaches with lemon juice. Stir gently. In a flameproof serving dish, melt the butter. Add the sugar and the peaches. Stir over fairly high heat for just a few moments, but do not cook. Pour the brandy into a heatproof ladle, ignite, and pour over the peaches. Serve immediately.

Yield: 4 servings.
Each serving contains:

Calories (Kcal): 107   Total fat (g): 3
Carbohydrates (g): 17   Protein (g): 1
Sodium (mg): 182   Cholesterol (mg): 117
Diabetic exchange: 1 fruit; 1 fat

Mexican Fresh Orange Dessert

Be sure to take the time to pull off all of the white parts under the orange skin for the sweetest taste.

4 large	sweet oranges, peeled, membrane removed	4 large
2 T	orange peel, grated	30 mL
4 t	fresh mint, finely chopped	20 mL
3 t	powdered sugar	15 mL
¼ C	light rum	60 mL

Alternate layers of orange slices sprinkled with the grated peel, chopped mint, powdered sugar, and rum in a glass or china bowl. Cover with plastic wrap and refrigerate for several hours. Stir before serving. Serve in dessert glasses.

Yield: 6 servings.
Each serving contains:
Calories (Kcal): 61
Carbohydrates (g): 15
Sodium (mg): 2
Diabetic exchange: 1 fruit

Total fat (g): 0
Protein (g): 1
Cholesterol (mg): 0

Hawaiian Grapes in Cream

The Hawaiians' love of sweets is moderated with cream in this unusual recipe. It's worth trying.

2 lbs.	white seedless grapes, stemmed	900 g
¾ C	dry Sherry	185 mL
4 C	low-fat frozen non-dairy whipped topping	1 L
3 T	sugar	45 mL
½ t	vanilla	3 mL
1 C	fat-free sour cream	250 mL

Put the grapes in a mixing bowl and pour the Sherry over them. Set aside for 2–3 hours to marinate. Drain off the Sherry and return the grapes to the bowl. In another bowl, combine the remaining ingredients. Fold into the grapes. Chill for at least 6 hours.

Yield: 8 servings.
Each serving contains:

Calories (Kcal): 199.6   Total fat (g): 0.5
Carbohydrates (g): 35.5   Protein (g): 1.7
Sodium (mg): 70   Cholesterol (mg): 2
Diabetic exchange: 3 fruit

Italian Strawberries and Balsamic Vinegar

This recipe is a surprising way to enjoy strawberries. Try this when they are at their ripest.

2 cups	strawberries, hulled and halved	500 mL
2 T	balsamic vinegar	30 mL

Place the strawberries in a bowl and carefully toss with the vinegar. Toss again just before serving.

Yield: 4 servings.
Each serving contains:

Calories (Kcal): 23	Total fat (g): 0
Carbohydrates (g): 6	Protein (g): 0
Sodium (mg): 1	Cholesterol (mg): 0
Diabetic exchange: free	

Italian Lemon Water Ice (Granita di Limone)

If you have an ice cream maker you can use it in this recipe. If not, the ice-cube tray technique works fine.

⅓ C	sugar	90 mL
2½ C	water	625 mL
1¼ C	fresh lemon juice	310 mL

In a saucepan, combine the sugar and the water. Stir to dissolve the sugar. Bring to a boil and boil for 5 minutes. Set aside until cool. Stir in the lemon juice. Pour into two metal ice cube trays and freeze until set.

Yield: 6 servings.
Each serving contains:
Calories (Kcal): 55.7   Total fat (g): 0
Carbohydrates (g): 15.5   Protein (g): 0.2
Sodium (mg): 4   Cholesterol (mg): 0
Diabetic exchange: 1 fruit

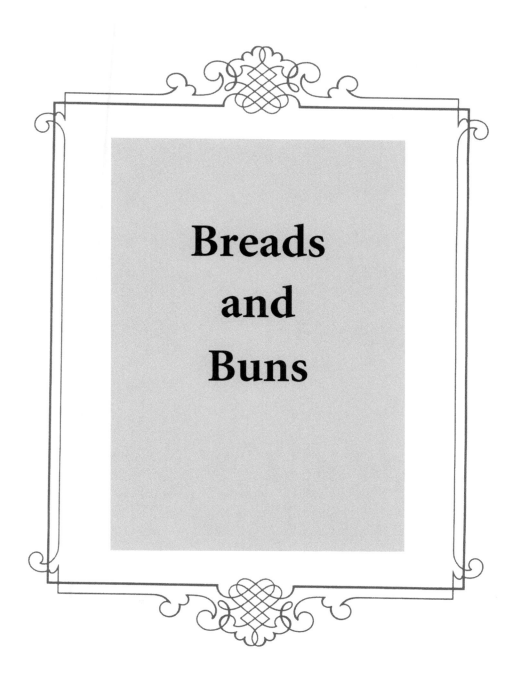

Breads
and
Buns

Haitian Sweet Potato Bread

No flour, but this "bread" is moist and smooth.

2 lbs.	sweet potatoes, peeled and cut in quarters	900 g
1 large	ripe banana, peeled and cut into 1-inch (3 cm) chunks	1 large
4 T	butter	60 mL
3 large	eggs or equivalent egg substitute, lightly beaten	3 large
¼ C	sugar	60 mL
¼ C	dark corn syrup	60 mL
½ C	lowfat 1% milk	125 g
½ C	evaporated milk	125 mL
½ t	vanilla extract	3 mL
¼ t	ground nutmeg	2 mL
¼ t	ground cinnamon	2 mL
¼ C	seedless raisins	60 mL

Bring a pot of water to a boil and drop in the sweet potatoes. Cook briskly until soft. Drain the sweet potatoes. Purée the banana and potatoes. Transfer to a mixing bowl. Beat in the butter and eggs. Add the remaining ingredients. Pour the batter into a well-greased 9 × 5 × 3-inch (23 × 12 × 8 cm) bread pan. Bake in a preheated 350° F (180° C) oven for 1½ hours. A cake tester in the center will come out clean. The top will be golden brown. Cool for about 5 minutes. Turn out onto a wire rack to cool completely.

Yield: 20 slices.
Each serving contains:

Calories (Kcal): 122

Total fat (g): 4

Carbohydrates (g): 21

Protein (g): 3

Sodium (mg): 169

Cholesterol (mg): 40

Diabetic exchange: 1 starch; 1 fat

Irish Barmbrack

This yeast bread rises twice and is wonderful with tea.

4 C	all-purpose flour	1 L
½ C	sugar	125 mL
½ t	ground cinnamon	3 mL
¼ t	ground allspice	2 mL
⅛ t	ground nutmeg	1 mL
½ t	salt	3 mL
1 env.	active baker's yeast	1 env.
1 C	lowfat 1% milk	250 mL
3 T	canola oil	45 mL
1 large	egg or equivalent egg substitute, lightly beaten	1 large
1 C	golden raisins	250 mL
½ C	currants	125 mL

Glaze frosting

1 T	confectioner's sugar	15 mL
2 T	boiling water	30 mL

In a mixing bowl, combine 1½ cups (325 mL) of the flour with the sugar, spices, salt, and yeast. Mix well. Combine the milk and oil in a small saucepan. Heat over low heat until very warm. Gradually add to the dry ingredient mixture. Beat for two minutes. Add the egg and ½ cup (125 mL) flour. Beat the milk mixture an additional two minutes. Stir in enough of the remaining flour to form a stiff dough. Turn out onto a lightly floured surface. Knead until smooth. Knead in the raisins and currants. Place in a lightly greased bowl and cover with a tea towel or plastic wrap. Set in a warm place free from drafts. Let the dough rise until double in bulk, approximately 1½ hours.

Punch down and form into a loaf. Place in a greased 9 × 5 × 3-inch (23 × 12 × 8 cm) pan. Cover with the towel and let rise in a warm place until again doubled in bulk, about 45 minutes. Bake in a preheated 400° F (200° C) oven for 50–60 minutes. The loaf should sound hollow when tapped.

Combine the sugar and water and brush the top of the hot loaf. Return to the oven for 3 more minutes. Remove loaf from pan and cool on wire rack.

Yield: 20 slices.
Each serving contains:

Calories (Kcal): 173
Carbohydrates (g): 34
Sodium (mg): 65
Diabetic exchange: 2 starch

Total fat (g): 3
Protein (g): 4
Cholesterol (mg): 11

Finnish Vilpuri Twist

Cardamom gives a traditional flavor to this coffee bread. This dough is a delight to work with.

5½ C	all-purpose flour	1325 mL
2 pkgs.	active baker's yeast	2 pkgs.
½ t	ground cardamom	3 mL
½ t	ground nutmeg	3 mL
2 C	lowfat 1% milk	500 mL
½ C	sugar	125 mL
¼ C	butter, margarine, or fat-free replacement	60 mL
1 t	salt	5 mL
1 large	egg, at room temperature, or egg substitute, lightly beaten	1 large
1 T	water	15 mL
1 large	egg, or equivalent egg substitute, lightly beaten	1 large

In a large mixing bowl combine 2½ cups (625 mL) flour with the yeast, cardamom, and nutmeg. In a saucepan, heat together the milk, sugar, butter, and salt just until warm. Add to the dry mixture. Add one egg. With an electric mixer, beat for a minute at a low speed, until thoroughly moistened, scraping the bowl constantly. Beat for three minutes at high speed. By hand, beat in enough of the remaining flour to make a stiff dough. Turn onto a floured work surface. Knead until smooth and elastic. Place in a greased bowl and turn once to grease the surface. Cover with a tea towel or plastic wrap. Let rise in a warm place until double in bulk (1–1½ hours).

Punch down. Divide into thirds and let rest for 10 minutes. On a lightly floured work surface, shape one-third of the dough into a rope at least 36 inches long. Form the dough rope into a circle with a six-inch (15 cm) overlap on the two ends closest to you. Holding the ends of the dough rope toward the center of the circle, twist together twice. Press the ends together and tuck under the center of the top of the circle, forming a pretzel-shaped roll. Place on a well-greased baking sheet. Repeat with the remaining dough to make three twists. Let each rise until almost double in bulk (30 to 45 minutes). Bake twists in a preheated 375° F (190° C) oven about 20 minutes. The breads will be light and will sound hollow when tapped. Beat the

GREAT INTERNATIONAL DIABETIC DESSERTS

remaining egg. Brush the egg mixture on the hot breads. Makes three loaves.

Yield: 60 slices.
Each serving contains:

Calories (Kcal): 62
Carbohydrates (g): 110
Sodium (mg): 50
Diabetic exchange: 1 starch

Total fat (g): 1
Protein (g): 2
Cholesterol (mg): 9

Irish Soda Bread

This traditional Irish quick bread is served in the late afternoon with tea. It all goes together easily, and you'll love having the smell of homemade bread baking in your home.

4 C	all-purpose flour, sifted	1 L
2 T	sugar	30 mL
1 t	active baker's yeast	5 mL
1 t	salt	5 mL
1 C	seedless raisins	250 mL
1 C	fat-free buttermilk*	250 mL
1 t	butter or equivalent butter substitute, softened	5 mL

*Or substitute with 1 C (250 mL) lowfat milk and 1 T (15 mL) vinegar.

Combine the first five ingredients in a mixing bowl and stir well. Make a well in the center. Add buttermilk or the buttermilk substitute. Stir until lightly but thoroughly blended. Use only enough buttermilk to make a stiff dough. Turn out onto a lightly floured work surface and knead only five times. Form into a ball and place on a lightly greased cookie sheet. Pat into an 8-inch (20 cm) circle, approximately 1½ inches (4 cm) thick.

With a floured knife, cut a large cross on top of the loaf. Spread the top of the loaf with butter. Bake in a preheated 375° F (165° C) oven 40 to 50 minutes or until golden. Serve hot, with jam or jelly.

Yield: 20 servings.
Each serving contains:

Calories (Kcal): 129   Total fat (g): 1
Carbohydrates (g): 28   Protein (g): 4
Sodium (mg): 121   Cholesterol (mg): 2
Diabetic exchange: 1 starch; 1 fruit

Irish Potato Scones

A substantial scone for afternoon tea.

3 T	butter, melted	45 mL
½ t	salt	3 mL
1 C	mashed potatoes, cold	250 mL
½ C	rolled oats	125 mL
½ t	baking powder	3 mL

Add the butter and salt to the mashed potatoes. Add the rolled oats and baking powder. Turn onto a floured work surface and add enough flour to make a stiff dough. Roll the dough out thick to the size of a saucer approximately 7½ inches (19 cm) in diameter. Cut it into wedges. Prick the top of each wedge with a fork and score it into quarters without cutting all the way through. Cook them on a hot griddle for 3–4 minutes each side. Serve hot.

Yield: 6 servings.
Each serving contains:
Calories (Kcal): 85   Total fat (g): 6
Carbohydrates (g): 7   Protein (g): 1
Sodium (mg): 335   Cholesterol (mg): 15
Diabetic exchange: 1 fat; ½ fruit

Irish Buttermilk Scones

These make a lovely breakfast treat, or serve them with soup for dinner on cool nights.

2 t	baking powder	10 mL
1 C	buttermilk (see note)	250 mL
2½ C	flour	625 mL
1 t	salt	5 mL

Note: If you don't have buttermilk you can use 1 cup (250 mL) of milk plus a tablespoon (15 mL) of vinegar.

Put the baking powder in a small mixing bowl. Add a little buttermilk and mix well. In another bowl combine the flour and the rest of the buttermilk, using a wooden spoon. Add the baking powder mixture. Mix thoroughly. Prepare a work surface by liberally dusting it with flour. Roll the dough into a circle 1½ inches (4 cm) thick. Cut into 16 wedges. Put the wedges on lightly greased baking sheets. Bake in a preheated 400° F (200° C) oven for 15 minutes. The scones will be lightly browned. Serve hot with sugar-free jam or jelly, if desired.

Yield: 16 scones.
Each serving contains:

Calories (Kcal): 77
Carbohydrates (g): 16
Sodium (mg): 195
Diabetic exchange: 1 starch

Total fat (g): 0
Protein (g): 3
Cholesterol (mg): 1

Irish Tea Scones

Our friends Bobby and Annette Donovan love these scones better than any others. They stopped by one Sunday morning and were fans of these after just one bite.

2 C	all-purpose flour	500 mL
1 T	active baker's yeast	15 mL
½ t	salt	3 mL
1 T	sugar	15 mL
4 T	butter, margarine, or fat-free replacement	60 mL
2 medium	eggs or equivalent egg substitute	2 medium
⅓ C	lowfat 1% milk	80 mL
1 medium	egg or equivalent egg substitute, lightly beaten	1 medium
1 T	lowfat 1% milk	15 mL

Combine the first four ingredients in a mixing bowl and mix well. Cut in the butter, using two knives or a pastry blender. Make a well in this mixture. Beat together the two eggs and third-cup milk and add to the flour mixture. Mix lightly but thoroughly. Turn the dough out onto a lightly floured surface and knead for five minutes. Roll into a 9-inch (23 cm) circle approximately ¾ inch (2 cm) thick. Cut into 12 pie-shaped wedges. Place the wedges onto a greased baking sheet. Beat together the remaining egg and milk. Brush the tops of the scones with this mixture. Bake in a preheated 400° F (200° C) oven for 7 to 10 minutes. Split scones. Serve with jam or jelly made without sugar, if desired.

Yield: 12 scones.
Each serving contains:
Calories (Kcal): 138
Carbohydrates (g): 18
Sodium (mg): 148
Total fat (g): 5
Protein (g): 5
Cholesterol (mg): 64
Diabetic exchange: 1 starch; 1 fat

Italian Rosemary Raisin Buns

Most big supermarkets have fresh rosemary in the produce section. When you have fresh rosemary, make these buns. They are well worth the effort.

¾ C	raisins, heaping	185 mL
2½ C	warm water	625 mL
2 envs.	active dry yeast	2 envs.
2 T	sugar	30 mL
2 T	olive oil	30 mL
3¾ C	flour	935 mL
1 t	salt	5 mL
2 T	olive oil	15 mL
2 t	rosemary sprigs, fresh, chopped	10 mL

Put the raisins in a small bowl and pour the warm water over them. Stir to combine and set aside for 20 minutes. Drain the raisins saving 1¼ cup (310 mL) of the raisin water to be used now and save the rest of the raisin water to use later as a glaze. In a small saucepan, warm the 1¼ cups (310 mL) in a small saucepan to about 105°–115° F (41°– 43° C) . Combine this heated water with the yeast in a large mixing bowl. Set aside for 10 minutes. The yeast should bubble, proof, and become creamy. Stir in the sugar and 2 T (30 mL) of olive oil. Stir in the salt. Add the flour gradually, mixing until the dough is no longer sticky. Turn onto a lightly floured work surface and knead until smooth and elastic.

Place the dough in an oiled bowl, cover with a tea towel or plastic wrap, and set to rise in a warm, draft-free place for an hour or until doubled in size.

Put the remaining 2 T (30 mL) of olive oil in a small frying pan and sauté the rosemary leaves and the drained raisins. Stir constantly. Cool. The raisins will be plump.

Punch down the dough and turn onto a lightly floured work surface. Shape the dough into a large rectangle. Sprinkle the rosemary mixture over the dough and roll up, jelly-roll style. Cover with a tea towel or plastic wrap for 10 minutes.

Shape the dough into 16 balls. Place the balls on lightly oiled cookie sheets. Cover with the towel and let rise for a second time for about an hour.

With a fork, prick a cross on the top of each bun. Reshape the buns into balls with your fingers, if needed. Brush on a glaze of reserved raisin water.

Cover with a towel again while the oven preheats to 400° F (200° C) . Bake for 15–20 minutes. Buns will be golden. Remove to racks to cool.

Yield: 16 servings.
Each serving contains:

Calories (Kcal): 168	Total fat (g): 4
Carbohydrates (g): 30	Protein (g): 4
Sodium (mg): 137	Cholesterol (mg): 0

Diabetic exchange: 1 starch; 1 fruit

Irish Currant Buns

A box of hot-roll mix makes these buns easy to make.

Buns

1 pkg. (6 oz.)	hot-roll mix	1 pkg. (120 g)
¼ C	warm water	60 mL
2 T	canola oil	30 mL
4 T	currants	60 mL
1 large	egg or equivalent egg substitute, lightly beaten	1 large
¼ C	sugar	60 mL
1 t	ground cinnamon	5 mL
½ t	nutmeg	3 mL

Glaze

1 large	egg yolk	1 large
1 T	lowfat 1% milk	15 mL

In a large mixing bowl, dissolve the yeast from the hot-roll mix in warm water. Add the oil and currants and mix well. Add the egg and stir to combine. Add the flour mixture from the hot-roll mix and the sugar and spices. Stir well. Cover with a tea towel or plastic wrap. Place the bowl in a warm place without drafts until the dough rises to double its bulk, about 45 minutes. Punch down the dough. Turn it out onto a floured surface. Knead it until it is no longer sticky, adding flour if needed. Divide into 12 balls of equal size. Place them next to one another in a greased 9 × 9-inch (23 × 23 cm) square pan. Cover with a towel or plastic wrap and let rise again in a warm place until double in volume.

Beat together the egg yolk and milk. Brush the dough with this egg mixture. Preheat the oven to 375 °F (190° C). Bake 15 minutes. Cool.

Yield: 12 buns.
Each serving contains:

Calories (Kcal): 62
Carbohydrates (g): 17
Sodium (mg): 101
Diabetic exchange: 1 starch

Total fat (g): 3
Protein (g): 2
Cholesterol (mg): 35

Italian Lemon Buns

These are light and flavorful. Perfect with espresso or fancy coffee.

¾ C	lowfat 1% milk	185 mL
2 envs.	active baker's yeast	2 envs. (14 g)
3½ C	flour	875 mL
¼ C	sugar	60 mL
1 t	salt	5 mL
⅓ C	olive oil	80 mL
2 large	eggs or equivalent egg substitute, lightly beaten	2 large
2 t	lemon peel, grated	10 mL
1 t	lemon extract	5 mL
1 t	vanilla extract	5 mL
1 large	egg white	1 large

Put the yeast into a small bowl. Heat the milk in a small saucepan to 105°–115°F (41°– 43° C). Pour over the yeast. Stir. Let stand for 10 minutes. The yeast should bubble and become creamy. Add ½ cup (125 mL) of the flour. Stir. Cover with a tea towel or plastic wrap. Set in a warm, draft-free place for 20 minutes. The mixture should double. Place the remaining flour, sugar, and salt into a large mixing bowl. Stir in the yeast mixture, olive oil, eggs, lemon peel, and extracts. Knead on a lightly floured work surface until smooth, adding more flour if needed. The dough inside will stay sticky. Place the dough in a lightly oiled bowl, cover with a tea towel or plastic wrap, and let rise for 1–2 hours, until doubled. Turn the dough out onto the lightly floured work surface and cut into 24 pieces. Roll each into a ball. Place them on lightly oiled cookie sheets. Cover with a tea towel or plastic wrap and let rise one hour, until doubled. Glaze each of the buns with the beaten egg white. Bake in a preheated 325° F (165° C) oven for 10 minutes. The buns should be golden and not too brown on the bottom. Remove to racks to cool.

Yield: 24 buns.
Each serving contains:

Calories (Kcal): 144	Total fat (g): 4
Carbohydrates (g): 17	Protein (g): 3
Sodium (mg): 101	Cholesterol (mg): 18

Diabetic exchange: 1 starch; 1 fat

Spanish French Toast Torrijas

French toast is a favorite Spanish dessert.

1 C	lowfat 1% milk	250 mL
½ t	cinnamon	3 mL
8 slices	white bread	8 slices
2 large	eggs or equivalent egg substitute, lightly beaten	2 large
dollop	fruit jam	dollop

Mix together milk and cinnamon in a shallow bowl. Briefly soak each slice of bread in the cinnamon milk, then dip in the beaten egg or egg substitute. Fry until brown in a hot griddle or frying pan sprayed with nonstick cooking spray. Serve immediately with jam.

Yield: 8 servings.
Each serving contains:

Calories (Kcal): 98

Carbohydrates (g): 14

Sodium (mg): 166

Diabetic exchange: 1 starch

Total fat (g): 3

Protein (g): 5

Cholesterol (mg): 55

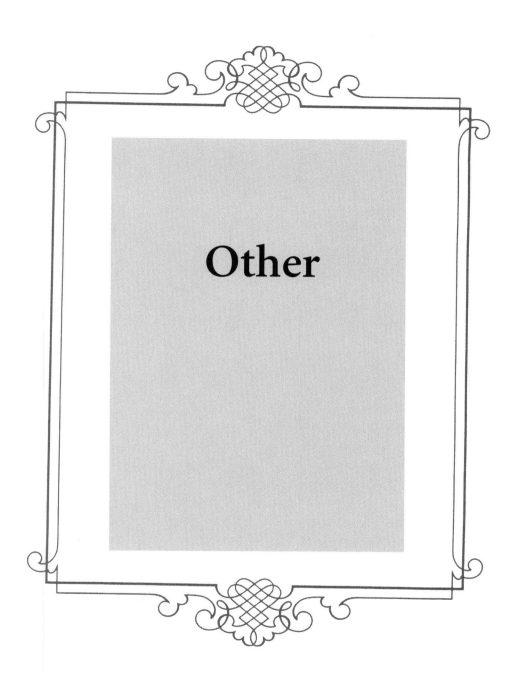

Other

Hungarian Baba au Rum

Make this the day before serving. It needs to age for 24 hours.

½ C	lowfat 1% milk	125 mL
2 T	butter, margarine, or fat-free butter and oil replacement	30 mL
2 T	canola oil	30 mL
1 t	salt	5 mL
¼ C	granulated sugar	60 mL
1 pkg.	active baker's yeast	1 pkg.
¼ C	warm water	60 mL
2 large	eggs or equivalent egg substitute, beaten	2 large
½ t	lemon peel, grated	3 mL
2¼ C	all-purpose flour	560 mL
½ C	water	125 mL
¼ C	molasses	60 mL
½ C	rum	125 mL

In a saucepan, scald the milk; add the butter, oil, salt, and ¼ cup (60 mL) granulated sugar until melted. Cool to lukewarm.

Dissolve the yeast in warm water. Add to the lukewarm milk and mix well. Stir in the beaten eggs and lemon peel. Add the flour and beat until smooth. Cover; let rise for five hours. Beat down and knead until smooth and elastic. Turn into a greased tube pan or baba mold. Let dough rise uncovered for another 30 minutes. Bake in a preheated 425°F (220° C) oven 20 minutes. Remove from pan at once to a cooling rack and then to a serving dish when cool.

In a heavy saucepan bring to a boil the water and molasses. Boil rapidly for 10 minutes. Cool slightly, add the rum, and stir well. Carefully spoon the rum sauce over the cake slowly, so that the sauce soaks into the cake. Cover tightly with aluminum foil and store for 24 hours before serving.

Yield: 16 servings.
Each serving contains:

Calories (Kcal): 148	Total fat (g): 4
Carbohydrates (g): 21	Protein (g): 3
Sodium (mg): 162	Cholesterol (mg): 31

Diabetic exchange: 1 starch; 1 fat

Polish Cottage-Cheese and Pear Snacks

This is a very fast dessert to make because the "cake" is actually pancakes. My friend Lois Arnold, who told me she doesn't like sponge cake, loved it.

1 can (10 oz.)	pear halves in juice	1 can (450 g)
1 C	white flour	250 mL
½ t	baking soda	3 mL
¼ t	salt	2 mL
1 T	granulated sugar	15 mL
1 whole	egg, beaten	1 whole
1 C	lowfat 1% milk	250 mL
1 T	vinegar	15 mL
2 C	lowfat small curd cottage cheese	500 mL

Drain the pear halves. Combine the flour, baking soda, salt, and sugar in a mixing bowl. Blend egg, milk, and vinegar in a small bowl. Add the milk mixture to the flour mixture and beat until smooth. Heat a skillet or griddle sprayed with nonstick spray until it is hot enough for a bead of water dropped on the surface to dance. Ladle enough batter onto the hot surface to make a small pancake. Cook until the top is covered with bubbles. Turn and cook on the other side. Repeat, using the remaining batter. Stack the pancakes, alternating each with a layer of cottage cheese. Arrange the pear quarters, fan-shaped, on top of the stack. Cut into wedges.

Yield: 8 servings.
Each serving contains:
Calories (Kcal): 166   Total fat (g): 10
Carbohydrates (g): 11   Protein (g): 7
Sodium (mg): 125   Cholesterol (mg): 177
Diabetic exchange: 1 fruit; 1 high-fat meat

Irish Shrove Tuesday Pancakes

Because eggs and milk were not used during Lent, traditionally in Ireland any eggs or milk in the house were made into pancakes for Shrove Tuesday, the day before Ash Wednesday.

2 C	all-purpose flour, sifted	500 mL
2 t	baking soda	10 mL
2 t	sugar	10 mL
½ t	salt	3 mL
2 medium	eggs or equivalent egg substitute, lightly beaten	3 medium
3 T	canola oil	45 mL
2 C	fat-free buttermilk*	500 mL

Sift the dry ingredients together into a mixing bowl. Beat the eggs, oil, and buttermilk together. Add the wet ingredients to the dry ones. Combine thoroughly but don't overmix; allow small lumps to remain. Heat a lightly oiled frying pan or griddle until a drop of water dances on it. Pour batter, ⅓ cup (80 mL) at a time, onto the griddle and cook until golden on the bottom and evenly covered with bubbles on the top. Turn and finish cooking on the other side.

*Or substitute with 2 C (500 mL) lowfat 1% milk, mixed with 2 T (30 mL) of vinegar.

Yield: 14 pancakes.
Each serving contains:
Calories (Kcal): 116   Total fat (g): 4
Carbohydrates (g): 16   Protein (g): 4
Sodium (mg): 297   Cholesterol (mg): 32
Diabetic exchange: 1 starch; 1 fat

French Baked Cherry Pancake

Whenever I see mountains of fresh cherries in the market I think of this recipe. I hope you'll love it, too.

1½ lbs.	black cherries, pitted	680 g
4 large	eggs or equivalent egg substitute, lightly beaten	4 large
1 pinch	salt	1 pinch
¼ C	sugar	60 mL
½ C	flour	125 mL
4 T	butter, margarine, or fat-free replacement	60 mL
1 C	lowfat 1% milk	225 mL
6 dollops	low-fat frozen non-dairy whipped topping (optional)	6 dollops

Put the cherries in a well-greased wide and shallow ovenproof dish. In a mixing bowl mix the eggs, salt, and sugar. Add the flour and beat well. Melt half the butter and beat it into the batter. Beat in the milk. Pour the batter over the cherries. Dot with the remaining butter. Bake in a preheated 400° F (200° C) oven for 35–40 minutes. The pancake is done when the batter is set. Serve hot or cold. Garnish with a dollop of whipped topping, if desired.

Yield: 12 servings.
Each serving contains:

Calories (Kcal): 128	Total fat (g): 6
Carbohydrates (g): 16	Protein (g): 4
Sodium (mg): 82	Cholesterol (mg): 82

Diabetic exchange: 1 starch; 1 fruit

Russian Dessert Pancakes

These are a staple on menus in Moscow. The batter can be made the day before and the pancakes before you begin to serve dinner.

1 C	all-purpose flour	250 mL
2 C	lowfat 1% milk	500 mL
2 large	egg yolks	2 large
2 T	sugar	30 mL
¼ t	salt	2 mL
2 large	egg whites	2 large
2 T	butter, margarine, or fat-free replacement, melted	30 mL
½ C	all-fruit blueberry (or other berry) jam	125 mL

Put the flour in a large mixing bowl and beat in the milk half a cup at a time. Then beat in the egg yolks, sugar, salt, and butter. When thoroughly combined, set the batter aside in a cool (not cold) place for at least three hours.

Before making the pancakes, beat the egg whites until they form stiff peaks. Use a rubber spatula to fold them into the batter. Preheat the oven to 250° F (120° C). Lightly coat a 5–6 inch (12–15 cm) crepe pan or skillet with a nonstick cooking spray. Pour in ½ cup (125 mL) of batter, tilting the pan to spread evenly. Fry over moderate heat for about three minutes on each side. The pancakes should be golden. Slide the pancake onto an oven-proof platter and keep warm in the oven while you fry the remaining pancakes similarly. Serve on heated dessert plates. Garnish with berry preserves.

Yield: 10 servings.
Each serving contains:

Calories (Kcal): 151	Total fat (g): 4
Carbohydrates (g): 24	Protein (g): 4
Sodium (mg): 114	Cholesterol (mg): 51

Diabetic exchange: 1 fruit; ½ lowfat milk; ½ fat

Mehren Pletzlach

A traditional Passover treat from Eastern Europe.

2 lbs.	carrots, cleaned, scraped, and shredded fine	900 g
¼ C	sugar	60 mL
1¾ t	ginger, powdered	9 mL
2 T	lemon juice, fresh	30 mL
1½ C	almonds, coarsely ground (optional)	375 mL
1 T	granulated sugar	15 mL

Put the carrots in a large saucepan. Stir in the sugar. Barely cover with water and bring to a boil. Cook over very low heat until the sugar is completely dissolved. Add the ginger and lemon juice; gently simmer until all the moisture has evaporated. (This may take a few hours.) Add chopped nuts, if desired. Sprinkle the granulated sugar on a work surface. Spread the mixture on top of the sugar to a ¾-inch (2 cm) thickness. Smooth with a spatula and tidy the edges. Mark into squares and cool. Roll each square into a ball. (Makes 40 balls.)

Yield: 40 servings.
Each serving contains:
Calories (Kcal): 16   Total fat (g): 0
Carbohydrates (g): 4   Protein (g): 0
Sodium (mg): 8   Cholesterol (mg): 0
Diabetic exchange: free

Dutch Fritters

An absolute necessity for Dutch settlers in New York to celebrate the coming of the new year.

3¼ C	flour	875 mL
2 envs.	yeast	2 envs.
1 C	lowfat 1% milk	250 mL
⅓ C	sugar	80 mL
¼ C	butter	60 mL
1 t	salt	5 mL
1 t	vanilla extract	5 mL
2 large	eggs or equivalent egg substitute	2 large
3 large	egg yolks	3 large
½ C	raisins	125 mL
	vegetable shortening for frying	

In a mixing bowl, combine 2 cups of the flour and the yeast. In a saucepan, heat the milk, sugar, butter, and salt until warm (about 115° F, or 45° C). Stir constantly. Add the vanilla extract and mix well. Pour onto the flour mixture. Mix well. Mix in the eggs and extra yolks. Beat at high speed for three minutes. Mix in the rest of the flour and the raisins. Cover with a tea towel or plastic wrap and set in a warm place to rise until double in bulk (about 30 minutes). Carefully drop into shortening that has been heated to 375° F (190° C). Fry for about three minutes, turning to brown evenly. Drain on paper toweling.

Yield: 36 fritters.
Each serving contains:
Calories (Kcal): 80
Carbohydrates (g): 13
Sodium (mg): 80
Diabetic exchange: 1 starch

Total fat (g): 2
Protein (g): 2
Cholesterol (mg): 33

West African Banana Fritters

A quick dessert with a lot of flavor.

½ C	flour	125 mL
3 T	sugar	45 mL
3 whole	eggs, or equivalent egg substitute	3 whole
1 C	low-fat 1% milk	250 mL
1 pound	ripe bananas (4 or 5, minimum)	450 g
	vegetable oil for deep frying	

In a mixing bowl, combine the flour and sugar using a wire whisk. Beat in the eggs one at a time. Slowly beat in the milk. Keep beating until the batter is very smooth. Add the bananas and mix well. Let stand while heating the oil.

In a large, heavy saucepan, pour in oil to a depth of 2 to 3 inches (5 to 7.5 cm). Heat the oil to 375° F (195° C). Fry the fritters ¼ cup (60 mL) at a time. They will spread to an oblong shape. Turn them until they are a rich, golden color on both sides. Drain on paper towels. Serve warm.

Yield: 20 fritters.
Each fritter contains:

Calories (Kcal): 67.9   Total fat (g): 2.4
Carbohydrates (g): 10.2   Protein (g): 1.9
Sodium (mg): 16   Cholesterol (mg): 32
Diabetic exchange: ½ starch;½ fat

Exchange Lists for Meal Planning

Y ou can make a difference in your blood glucose control through your food choices. You do not need special foods. In fact, the foods that are good for you are good for everyone.

If you have diabetes, it is important to eat about the same amount of food at the same time each day. Regardless of what your blood glucose level is, try not to skip meals or snacks. Skipping meals and snacks may lead to large swings in blood glucose levels.

To keep your blood glucose levels near normal, you need to balance the food you eat with the insulin your body makes or gets by injection and with your physical activities. Blood glucose monitoring gives you information to help you with this balancing act. Near-normal blood glucose levels help you feel better. And they may reduce or prevent the complications of diabetes.

The number of calories you need depends on your size, age, and activity level. If you are an adult, eating the right number of calories can help you reach and stay at a reasonable weight. Children and adolescents must eat enough calories so they grow and develop normally. Don't limit their calories to try to control blood glucose levels. Instead, adjust their insulin to cover the calories they need.

Of course, everyone needs to eat nutritious foods. Our good health depends on eating a variety of foods that contain the right amounts of carbohydrate, protein, fat, vitamins, minerals, fiber, and water.

What Are Carbohydrate, Protein, and Fat?

Carbohydrate, protein, and fat are found in the food you eat. They supply your body with energy, or calories. Your body needs insulin to use this energy. Insulin is made in the pancreas. If you have diabetes, either your pancreas is no longer making insulin or your body can't use the insulin it is making. In either case, your blood glucose levels are not normal.

Carbohydrate. Starch and sugar in foods are carbohydrates. Starch is in breads, pasta, cereals, potatoes, peas, beans, and lentils. Naturally present sugars are in fruits, milk, and vegetables. Added sugars are in desserts, candy, jams, and syrups. All of these carbohydrates provide 4 calories per gram and can affect your blood glucose levels.

When you eat carbohydrates, they turn into glucose and travel in your bloodstream. Insulin helps the glucose enter the cells, where it can be used for energy or stored. Eating the same amount of carbohydrate daily at meals and snacks helps you control your blood glucose levels.

Protein. Protein is in meats, poultry, fish, milk and other dairy products, eggs, and beans, peas, and lentils. Starches and vegetables also have small amounts of protein.

The body uses protein for growth, maintenance, and energy. Protein has 4 calories of energy per gram. Again, your body needs insulin to use the protein you eat.

Fat. Fat is in margarine, butter, oils, salad dressings, nuts, seeds, milk, cheese, meat, fish, poultry, snack foods, ice cream, and desserts.

There are different types of fat: monounsaturated, polyunsaturated, and saturated. Everyone should eat less of the saturated fats found in meats, dairy products, coconut, palm or palm kernel oil, and hardened shortenings. Saturated fats can raise your blood levels of cholesterol. The fats that are best are the monounsaturated fats found in canola oil, olive oil, nuts, and avocado. The polyunsaturated fats found in corn oil, soybean oil, or sunflower oil are also good choices.

After you eat fat, it travels in your bloodstream. You need insulin to store fat in the cells of your body. Fats are used for energy. In fact, fats have 9 calories per gram, more than two times the calories you get from carbohydrate and protein.

What Else Do I Need to Know?
Vitamins and Minerals. Most foods in the exchange lists are good sources of vitamins and minerals. If you eat a variety of these foods you probably do not need a vitamin or mineral supplement.

Salt or Sodium. High blood pressure may be made worse by eating too much sodium (salt and salty foods). Try to use less salt in cooking and at the table.

In the lists, foods that are high in sodium (400 milligrams or more of sodium per exchange) have a salt shaker symbol (✒).

Alcohol. You may have an alcoholic drink occasionally. If you take insulin or a diabetes pill, be sure to eat food with your drink. Ask your dietitian about a safe amount of alcohol for you and how to work it into your meal plan.

How Do I Know What to Eat and When?
You and your dietitian will work out a meal plan to get the right balance between your food, medication, and exercise.

The lists of food choices (exchange lists) can help you make interesting and healthy food choices. Exchange lists and a meal plan help you know what to eat, how much to eat, and when to eat.

There are three main groups—the Carbohydrate group, the Meat and Meat Substitute group (protein), and the Fat group. Starch, fruit, milk, other carbohydrates, and vegetables are in the Carbohydrate group. The Meat and Meat Substitute group is divided into very lean, lean, medium-fat, and high-fat foods. You can see at a glance which are the lower-fat choices. Foods in the Fat group—monounsaturated, polyunsaturated, and saturated—have very small serving sizes.

What Are Exchange Lists?
Exchange lists are foods listed together because they are alike. Each serving of a food has about the same amount of carbohydrate, protein, fat, and calories as the other foods on that list. That is why any food on a list can be "exchanged," or traded, for any other food on the same list. For example, you can trade the slice of

bread you might eat for breakfast for one-half cup of cooked cereal. Each of these foods equals one starch choice.

Exchange Lists

Foods are listed with their serving sizes, which are usually measured after cooking. When you begin, you should measure the size of each serving. This may help you learn to "eyeball" correct serving sizes.

The following chart shows the amount of nutrients in one serving from each list.

Groups/Lists	Carbohydrate (grams)	Protein (grams)	Fat (grams)	Calories
Carbohydrate Group				
Starch	15	3	1 or less	80
Fruit	15	—	—	60
Milk				
Skim	12	8	0–3	90
Low-fat	12	8	5	120
Whole	12	8	8	150
Other carbohydrates	15	varies	varies	varies
Vegetables	5	2	—	25
Meat and Meat Substitute Group				
Very lean	—	7	0–1	35
Lean	—	7	3	55
Medium-fat	—	7	5	75
High-fat	—	7	8	100
Fat Group	—	—	5	45

The exchange lists provide you with a lot of food choices (foods from the basic food groups, foods with added sugars, free foods, combination foods, and fast foods). This gives you variety in your meals. Several foods, such as beans, peas, and lentils, bacon, and peanut butter, are on two lists. This gives you flexibility in putting your meals together. Whenever you choose new foods or vary your meal plan, monitor your blood glucose to see how these different foods affect your blood glucose level.

Most foods in the Carbohydrate group have about the same amount of carbohydrate per serving. You can exchange starch, fruit, or milk choices in your meal plan. Vegetables are in this group but contain only about 5 grams of carbohydrate.

A Word about Food Labels

Exchange information is based on foods found in grocery stores. However, food companies often change the ingredients in their products. That is why you need to check the Nutrition Facts panel of the food label.

The Nutrition Facts tell you the number of calories and grams of carbohydrate, protein, and fat in one serving. Compare these numbers with the exchange information to see how many exchanges you will be eating. In this way, food labels can help you add foods to your meal plans.

Ask your dietitian to help you use food label information to plan your meals.

Getting Started!

See your dietitian regularly when you are first learning how to use your meal plan and the exchange lists. Your meal plan can be adjusted to fit changes in your lifestyle, such as work, school, vacation, or travel. Regular nutrition counseling can help you make positive changes in your eating habits.

Careful eating habits will help you feel better and be healthier, too. Best wishes and good eating with *Exchange Lists for Meal Planning*.

Starch List

Cereals, grains, pasta, breads, crackers, snacks, starchy vegetables, and cooked beans, peas, and lentils are starches. In general, one starch is:
- ½ cup of cereal, grain, pasta, or starchy vegetable,
- 1 ounce of a bread product, such as 1 slice of bread,
- ¾ to 1 ounce of most snack foods. (Some snack foods may also have added fat.)

Nutrition Tips

1. Most starch choices are good sources of B vitamins.
2. Foods made from whole grains are good sources of fiber.
3. Beans, peas, and lentils are a good source of protein and fiber.

Selection Tips

1. Choose starches made with little fat as often as you can.
2. Starchy vegetables prepared with fat count as one starch and one fat.
3. Bagels or muffins can be 2, 3, or 4 ounces in size, and can, therefore, count as 2, 3, or 4 starch choices. Check the size you eat.
4. Most of the serving sizes are measured after cooking.
5. Always check Nutrition Facts on the food label.

One starch exchange equals 15 grams carbohydrate, 3 grams protein, 0–1 grams fat, and 80 calories.

Bread

Bagel	½ (1 oz)	Hot dog or hamburger bun	½ (1 oz)
Bread, reduced-calorie	2 slices (1½ oz)	Pita, 6 in. across	½
		Raisin bread, unfrosted	1 slice (1 oz)
Bread, white, whole-wheat, pumpernickel, rye	1 slice (1 oz)	Roll, plain, small	1 (1 oz)
		Tortilla, corn, 6 in. across	1
Bread sticks, crisp, 4 in. long x ½ in.	2 (⅔ oz)	Tortilla, flour, 7–8 in. across	1
		Waffle, 4½ in. square, reduced-fat	1
English muffin	½		

Cereals and Grains

Bran cereals	½ cup
Bulgur	½ cup
Cereals	½ cup
Cereals, unsweetened, ready-to-eat	¾ cup
Cornmeal (dry)	3 Tbsp
Couscous	⅓ cup
Flour (dry)	3 Tbsp
Granola, low-fat	¼ cup
Grape-Nuts®	¼ cup
Grits	½ cup
Kasha	½ cup
Millet	¼ cup
Muesli	¼ cup
Oats	½ cup
Pasta	½ cup
Puffed cereal	1½ cups
Rice milk	½ cup
Rice, white or brown	⅓ cup
Shredded Wheat®	½ cup
Sugar-frosted cereal	½ cup
Wheat germ	3 Tbsp

Starchy Vegetables

Baked beans	⅓ cup
Corn	½ cup
Corn on cob, medium	1 (5 oz)
Mixed vegetables with corn, peas, or pasta	1 cup
Peas, green	½ cup
Plantain	½ cup
Potato, baked or boiled	1 small (3 oz)
Potato, mashed	½ cup
Squash, winter (acorn, butternut)	1 cup
Yam, sweet potato, plain	½ cup

Crackers and Snacks

Animal crackers	8
Graham crackers, 2½ in. square	3
Matzoh	¾ oz
Melba toast	4 slices
Oyster crackers	24
Popcorn (popped, no fat added or low-fat microwave)	3 cups
Pretzels	¾ oz
Rice cakes, 4 in. across	2
Saltine-type crackers	6
Snack chips, fat-free (tortilla, potato)	15–20 (¾ oz)
Whole-wheat crackers, no fat added	2–5 (¾ oz)

Beans, Peas, and Lentils

(*Count as 1 starch exchange, plus 1 very lean meat exchange.*)

Beans and peas (garbanzo, pinto, kidney, white, split, black-eyed)	½ cup
Lima beans	⅔ cup
Lentils	½ cup
Miso ◣	3 Tbsp

Starchy Foods Prepared with Fat

(*Count as 1 starch exchange, plus 1 fat exchange.*)

Biscuit, 2½ in. across	1
Chow mein noodles	½ cup
Corn bread, 2 in. cube	1 (2 oz)
Crackers, round butter type	6
Croutons	1 cup
French-fried potatoes	16–25 (3 oz)
Granola	¼ cup
Muffin, small	1 (1½ oz)
Pancake, 4 in. across	2
Popcorn, microwave	3 cups
Sandwich crackers, cheese or peanut butter filling	3
Stuffing, bread (prepared)	⅓ cup
Taco shell, 6 in. across	2
Waffle, 4½ in. square	1
Whole-wheat crackers, fat added	4–6 (1 oz)

◣ = 400 mg or more of sodium per exchange.

Starches often swell in cooking, so a small amount of uncooked starch will become a much larger amount of cooked food. The following table shows some of the changes.

Food (Starch Group)	Uncooked	Cooked
Oatmeal	3 Tbsp	½ cup
Cream of wheat	2 Tbsp	½ cup
Grits	3 Tbsp	½ cup
Rice	2 Tbsp	⅓ cup
Spaghetti	¼ cup	½ cup
Noodles	⅓ cup	½ cup
Macaroni	¼ cup	½ cup
Dried beans	¼ cup	½ cup
Dried peas	¼ cup	½ cup
Lentils	3 Tbsp	½ cup

Fruit List

Fresh, frozen, canned, and dried fruits and fruit juices are on this list. In general, one fruit exchange is:
- 1 small to medium fresh fruit,
- ½ cup of canned or fresh fruit or fruit juice,
- ¼ cup of dried fruit.

Nutrition Tips

1. Fresh, frozen, and dried fruits have about 2 grams of fiber per choice. Fruit juices contain very little fiber.
2. Citrus fruits, berries, and melons are good sources of vitamin C.

Selection Tips

1. Count ½ cup cranberries or rhubarb sweetened with sugar substitutes as free foods.
2. Read the Nutrition Facts on the food label. If one serving has more than 15 grams of carbohydrate, you will need to adjust the size of the serving you eat or drink.
3. Portion sizes for canned fruits are for the fruit and a small amount of juice.
4. Whole fruit is more filling than fruit juice and may be a better choice.
5. Food labels for fruits may contain the words "no sugar added" or "unsweetened." This means that no sucrose (table sugar) has been added.
6. Generally, fruit canned in extra light syrup has the same amount of carbohydrate per serving as the "no sugar added" or the juice pack. All canned fruits on the fruit list are based on one of these three types of pack.

One fruit exchange equals 15 grams carbohydrate and 60 calories. The weight includes skin, core, seeds, and rind.

Fruit	
Apple, unpeeled, small	1 (4 oz)
Applesauce, unsweetened	½ cup
Apples, dried	4 rings
Apricots, fresh	4 whole (5½ oz)
Apricots, dried	8 halves
Apricots, canned	½ cup
Banana, small	1 (4 oz)
Blackberries	¾ cup
Blueberries	¾ cup
Cantaloupe, small	⅓ melon (11 oz)
	or 1 cup cubes
Cherries, sweet, fresh	12 (3 oz)
Cherries, sweet, canned	½ cup
Dates	3
Figs, fresh	1½ large
	or 2 medium (3½ oz)
Figs, dried	1½
Fruit cocktail	½ cup
Grapefruit, large	½ (11 oz)
Grapefruit sections, canned	¾ cup
Grapes, small	17 (3 oz)
Honeydew melon	1 slice (10 oz)
	or 1 cup cubes
Kiwi	1 (3½ oz)
Mandarin oranges, canned	¾ cup
Mango, small	½ fruit (5½ oz)
	or ½ cup
Nectarine, small	1 (5 oz)

Orange, small	1 (6½ oz)
Papaya	½ fruit (8 oz)
	or 1 cup cubes
Peach, medium, fresh	1 (6 oz)
Peaches, canned	½ cup
Pear, large, fresh	½ (4 oz)
Pears, canned	½ cup
Pineapple, fresh	¾ cup
Pineapple, canned	½ cup
Plums, small	2 (5 oz)
Plums, canned	½ cup
Prunes, dried	3
Raisins	2 Tbsp
Raspberries	1 cup
Strawberries	1¼ cup whole berries
Tangerines, small	2 (8 oz)
Watermelon	1 slice (13½ oz)
	or 1¼ cup cubes

Fruit Juice

Apple juice/cider	½ cup
Cranberry juice cocktail	⅓ cup
Cranberry juice cocktail, reduced-calorie	1 cup
Fruit juice blends, 100% juice	⅓ cup
Grape juice	⅓ cup
Grapefruit juice	½ cup
Orange juice	½ cup
Pineapple juice	½ cup
Prune juice	⅓ cup

Milk List

Different types of milk and milk products are on this list. Cheeses are on the Meat list and cream and other dairy fats are on the Fat list. Based on the amount of fat they contain, milks are divided into skim/very low-fat milk, low-fat milk, and whole milk. One choice of these includes:

	Carbohydrate (grams)	Protein (grams)	Fat (grams)	Calories
Skim/very low-fat	12	8	0–3	90
Low-fat	12	8	5	120
Whole	12	8	8	150

Nutrition Tips

1. Milk and yogurt are good sources of calcium and protein. Check the food label.
2. The higher the fat content of milk and yogurt, the greater the amount of saturated fat and cholesterol. Choose lower-fat varieties.
3. For those who are lactose intolerant, look for lactose-reduced or lactose-free varieties of milk.

Selection Tips

1. One cup equals 8 fluid ounces or ½ pint.
2. Look for chocolate milk, frozen yogurt, and ice cream on the Other Carbohydrates list.
3. Nondairy creamers are on the Free Foods list.
4. Look for rice milk on the Starch list.

One milk exchange equals 12 grams carbohydrate and 8 grams protein.

Skim and Very Low-fat Milk
(0–3 grams fat per serving)

Skim milk	1 cup
½% milk	1 cup
1% milk	1 cup
Nonfat or low-fat buttermilk	1 cup
Evaporated skim milk	½ cup
Nonfat dry milk	⅓ cup dry
Plain nonfat yogurt	¾ cup
Nonfat or low-fat fruit-flavored yogurt sweetened with aspartame or with a nonnutritive sweetener	1 cup

Low-fat
(5 grams fat per serving)

2% milk	1 cup
Plain low-fat yogurt	¾ cup
Sweet acidophilus milk	1 cup

Whole Milk
(8 grams fat per serving)

Whole milk	1 cup
Evaporated whole milk	½ cup
Goat's milk	1 cup
Kefir	1 cup

Vegetable List

Vegetables that contain small amounts of carbohydrates and calories are on this list. Vegetables contain important nutrients. Try to eat at least 2 or 3 vegetable choices each day. In general, one vegetable exchange is:
- ½ cup of cooked vegetables or vegetable juice,
- 1 cup of raw vegetables.

If you eat 1 to 2 vegetable choices at a meal or snack, you do not have to count the calories or carbohydrates because they contain small amounts of these nutrients.

Nutrition Tips
1. Fresh and frozen vegetables have less added salt than canned vegetables. Drain and rinse canned vegetables if you want to remove some salt.
2. Choose more dark green and dark yellow vegetables, such as spinach, broccoli, romaine, carrots, chilies, and peppers.
3. Broccoli, brussels sprouts, cauliflower, greens, peppers, spinach, and tomatoes are good sources of vitamin C.
4. Vegetables contain 1 to 4 grams of fiber per serving.

Selection Tips
1. A one-cup portion of broccoli is a portion about the size of a lightbulb.
2. Canned vegetables and juices are available without added salt.
3. If you eat more than 3 cups of raw vegetables or 1½ cups of cooked vegetables at one meal, count them as 1 carbohydrate choice.
4. Starchy vegetables such as corn, peas, winter squash, and potatoes that contain larger amounts of calories and carbohydrates are on the Starch list.

One vegetable exchange equals 5 grams carbohydrate, 2 grams protein, 0 grams fat, and 25 calories.

Artichoke
Artichoke hearts
Asparagus
Beans (green, wax, Italian)
Bean sprouts
Beets
Broccoli
Brussels sprouts
Cabbage
Carrots
Cauliflower
Celery
Cucumber
Eggplant
Green onions or scallions
Greens (collard, kale, mustard, turnip)

Kohlrabi
Leeks
Mixed vegetables (without corn, peas, or pasta)
Mushrooms
Okra
Onions
Pea pods
Peppers (all varieties)
Radishes
Salad greens (endive, escarole, lettuce, romaine, spinach)
Sauerkraut ▰
Spinach

▰ = 400 mg or more sodium per exchange.

Summer squash
Tomato
Tomatoes, canned
Tomato sauce ◣
Tomato/vegetable juice ◣
Turnips

Water chestnuts
Watercress
Zucchini
   ◣ = 400 mg or more sodium per
      exchange.

Meat and Meat Substitutes List

Meat and meat substitutes that contain both protein and fat are on this list. In general, one meat exchange is:

- 1 ounce meat, fish, poultry, or cheese,
- ½ cup beans, peas, and lentils. Based on the amount of fat they contain, meats are divided into very lean, lean, medium-fat, and high-fat lists. This is done so you can see which ones contain the least amount of fat. One ounce (one exchange) of each of these includes:

	Carbohydrate (grams)	Protein (grams)	Fat (grams)	Calories
Very lean	0	7	0–1	35
Lean	0	7	3	55
Medium-fat	0	7	5	75
High-fat	0	7	8	100

Nutrition Tips

1. Choose very lean and lean meat choices whenever possible. Items from the high-fat group are high in saturated fat, cholesterol, and calories and can raise blood cholesterol levels.
2. Meats do not have any fiber.
3. Some processed meats, seafood, and soy products may contain carbohydrate when consumed in large amounts. Check the Nutrition Facts on the label to see if the amount is close to 15 grams. If so, count it as a carbohydrate choice as well as a meat choice.

Selection Tips

1. Weigh meat after cooking and removing bones and fat. Four ounces of raw meat is equal to 3 ounces of cooked meat. Some examples of meat portions are:
- 1 ounce cheese = 1 meat choice and is about the size of a one-inch cube
- 2 ounces meat = 2 meat choices, such as 1 small chicken leg or thigh or ½ cup cottage cheese or tuna
- 3 ounces meat = 3 meat choices and is about the size of a deck of cards, such as 1 medium pork chop, 1 small hamburger, ½ of a whole chicken breast, or 1 unbreaded fish fillet
2. Limit your choices from the high-fat group to three times per week or less.

3. Most grocery stores stock Select and Choice grades of meat. Select grades of meat are the leanest meats. Choice grades contain a moderate amount of fat, and Prime cuts of meat have the highest amount of fat. Restaurants usually serve Prime cuts of meat.
4. "Hamburger" may contain added seasoning and fat, but ground beef does not.
5. Read labels to find products that are low in fat and cholesterol (5 grams or less of fat per serving).
6. Peanut butter, in smaller amounts, is also found on the Fats list.
7. Bacon, in smaller amounts, is also found on the Fats list.

Meal Planning Tips
1. Bake, roast, broil, grill, poach, steam, or boil these foods rather than frying.
2. Place meat on a rack so the fat will drain off during cooking.
3. Use a nonstick spray and a nonstick pan to brown or fry foods.
4. Trim off visible fat before or after cooking.
5. If you add flour, bread crumbs, coating mixes, fat, or marinades when cooking, ask your dietitian how to count it in your meal plan.

Lean Meat and Substitutes List

One exchange equals 0 grams carbohydrate, 7 grams protein, 3 grams fat, and 55 calories.

One lean meat exchange is equal to any one of the following items.

Beef: USDA Select or Choice grades of lean beef trimmed of fat, such as round, sirloin, and flank steak; tenderloin; roast (rib, chuck, rump); steak (T-bone, porterhouse, cubed); ground round   1 oz

Pork: Lean pork, such as fresh ham; canned, cured, or boiled ham; Canadian bacon ➤ ; tenderloin, center loin chop   1 oz

Lamb: Roast, chop, leg   1 oz

Veal: Lean chop, roast   1 oz

Poultry: Chicken, turkey (dark meat, no skin), chicken (white meat, with skin), domestic duck or goose (well-drained of fat, no skin)   1 oz

Fish:
  Herring
  (uncreamed or smoked)   1 oz
  Oysters   6 medium

Salmon (fresh or canned),
  catfish   1 oz
  Sardines (canned)   2 medium
  Tuna (canned in oil, drained)   1 oz
Game: Goose (no skin), rabbit   1 oz
Cheese:
  4.5%-fat cottage cheese   ¼ cup
  Grated Parmesan   2 Tbsp
  Cheeses with 3 grams or less fat per ounce   1 oz
Other:
  Hot dogs with 3 grams or less fat per ounce ➤   1½ oz
  Processed sandwich meat with 3 grams or less fat per ounce, such as turkey pastrami or kielbasa   1 oz
  Liver, heart (high in cholesterol)   1 oz

High-Fat Meat and Substitutes List

One exchange equals 0 grams carbohydrate, 7 grams protein, 8 grams fat, and 100 calories.

Remember that these items are high in saturated fat, cholesterol, and calories and may raise blood cholesterol levels if eaten on a regular basis.

One high-fat meat exchange is equal to any one of the following items.

Pork: Spareribs, ground pork, pork sausage   1 oz

Cheese: All regular cheeses, such as American ➤, Cheddar, Monterey Jack, Swiss   1 oz

Other: Processed sandwich meats with 8 grams or less fat per ounce, such as bologna, pimento loaf, salami   1 oz

Sausage, such as bratwurst, Italian, knockwurst, Polish, smoked   1 oz

Hot dog (turkey or chicken) ➤   1 (10/lb)

Bacon   3 slices (20 slices/lb)

Count as one high-fat meat plus one fat exchange.

Hot dog (beef, pork, or combination) ➤   1 (10/lb)

Peanut butter (contains unsaturated fat)   2 Tbsp

➤ = 400 mg or more sodium per exchange.

Fat List

Fats are divided into three groups, based on the main type of fat they contain: monounsaturated, polyunsaturated, and saturated. Small amounts of monounsaturated and polyunsaturated fats in the foods we eat are linked with good health benefits. Saturated fats are linked with heart disease and cancer. In general, one fat exchange is:

- 1 teaspoon of regular margarine or vegetable oil,
- 1 tablespoon of regular salad dressings.

Nutrition Tips

1. All fats are high in calories. Limit serving sizes for good nutrition and health.
2. Nuts and seeds contain small amounts of fiber, protein, and magnesium.
3. If blood pressure is a concern, choose fats in the unsalted form to help lower sodium intake, such as unsalted peanuts.

Selection Tips

1. Check the Nutrition Facts on food labels for serving sizes. One fat exchange is based on a serving size containing 5 grams of fat.
2. When selecting regular margarines, choose those with liquid vegetable oil as the first ingredient. Soft margarines are not as saturated as stick margarines. Soft margarines are healthier choices. Avoid those listing hydrogenated or partially hydrogenated fat as the first ingredient.
3. When selecting low-fat margarines, look for liquid vegetable oil as the second ingredient. Water is usually the first ingredient.

4. When used in smaller amounts, bacon and peanut butter are counted as fat choices. When used in larger amounts, they are counted as high-fat meat choices.
5. Fat-free salad dressings are on the Free Foods list.
6. See the Free Foods list for nondairy coffee creamers, whipped topping, and fat-free products, such as margarines, salad dressings, mayonnaise, sour cream, cream cheese, and nonstick cooking spray.

Monounsaturated Fats List

(One fat exchange equals 5 grams fat and 45 calories.)

Avocado, medium	⅛ (1 oz)
Oil (canola, olive, peanut)	1 tsp
Olives: ripe (black)	8 large
green, stuffed ✎	10 large
Nuts	
almonds, cashews	6 nuts
mixed (50% peanuts)	6 nuts
peanuts	10 nuts
pecans	4 halves
Peanut butter, smooth or crunchy	2 tsp
Sesame seeds	1 Tbsp
Tahini paste	2 tsp

Polyunsaturated Fats List

(One fat exchange equals 5 grams fat and 45 calories.)

Margarine: stick, tub, or squeeze	1 tsp
lower-fat	
(30% to 50% vegetable oil)	1 Tbsp
Mayonnaise: regular	1 tsp
reduced-fat	1 Tbsp
Nuts, walnuts, English	4 halves
Oil (corn, safflower, soybean)	1 tsp
Salad dressing: regular ✎	1 Tbsp
reduced-fat	2 Tbsp

Miracle Whip Salad Dressing®:

regular	2 tsp
reduced-fat	1 Tbsp
Seeds: pumpkin, sunflower	1 Tbsp

Saturated Fats List*

(One fat exchange equals 5 grams fat and 45 calories.)

Bacon, cooked	1 slice (20 slices/lb)
Bacon, grease	1 tsp
Butter: stick	1 tsp
whipped	2 tsp
reduced-fat	1 Tbsp
Chitterlings, boiled	2 Tbsp (½ oz)
Coconut, sweetened, shredded	2 Tbsp
Cream, half and half	2 Tbsp
Cream cheese: regular	1 Tbsp (½ oz)
reduced-fat	2 Tbsp (1 oz)
Fatback or salt pork, see below	
Shortening or lard	1 tsp
Sour cream: regular	2 Tbsp
reduced-fat	3 Tbsp

Use a piece 1 in.×1 in.×¼ in. if you plan to eat the fatback cooked with vegetables. Use a piece 2 in. x 1 in. x ½ in. when eating only the vegetables with the fatback removed.

*Saturated fats can raise blood cholesterol levels.

Free Foods List

A *free food* is any food or drink that contains less than 20 calories or less than 5 grams of carbohydrate per serving. Foods with a serving size listed should be limited to three servings per day. Be sure to spread them out throughout the day. If you eat all three servings at one time, it could affect your blood glucose level. Foods listed without a serving size may be eaten as often as you like.

Fat-free or Reduced-fat Foods

Cream cheese, fat-free	1 Tbsp
Creamers, nondairy, liquid	1 Tbsp
Creamers, nondairy, powdered	2 tsp
Mayonnaise, fat-free	1 Tbsp
Mayonnaise, reduced-fat	1 tsp
Margarine, fat-free	4 Tbsp
Margarine, reduced-fat	1 tsp
Miracle Whip®, nonfat	1 Tbsp
Miracle Whip®, reduced-fat	1 tsp
Nonstick cooking spray	
Salad dressing, fat-free	1 Tbsp
Salad dressing, fat-free, Italian	2 Tbsp
Salsa	¼ cup
Sour cream, fat-free, reduced-fat	1 Tbsp
Whipped topping, regular or light	2 Tbsp

Sugar-free or Low-sugar Foods

Candy, hard, sugar-free	1 candy
Gelatin dessert, sugar-free	
Gelatin, unflavored	
Gum, sugar-free	
Jam or jelly, low-sugar or light	2 tsp
Sugar substitutes	
Syrup, sugar-free	2 Tbsp

Sugar substitutes, alternatives, or replacements that are approved by the Food and Drug Administration (FDA) are safe to use. Common brand names include: Equal® (aspartame), Sprinkle Sweet® (saccharin), Sweet One® (acesulfame K), Sweet-10® (saccharin), Sugar Twin®, (saccharin), Sweet 'n Low® (saccharin)

Drinks

Bouillon, broth, consommé ⬥	
Bouillon or broth, low-sodium	
Carbonated or mineral water	
Club soda	
Cocoa powder, unsweetened	1 Tbsp
Coffee	
Diet soft drinks, sugar-free	
Drink mixes, sugar-free	
Tea	
Tonic water, sugar-free	

Condiments

Catsup	1 Tbsp
Horseradish	
Lemon juice	
Lime juice	
Mustard	
Pickles, dill ⬥	1½ large
Soy sauce, regular or light ⬥	
Taco sauce	1 Tbsp
Vinegar	

Seasonings

Be careful with seasonings that contain sodium or are salts, such as garlic or celery salt, and lemon pepper.

Flavoring extracts
Garlic
Herbs, fresh or dried
Pimento
Spices
Tabasco® or hot pepper sauce
Wine, used in cooking
Worcestershire sauce

⬥ = 400 mg or more of sodium per choice.

Index